Active Middle Ear Implants

Advances in Oto-Rhino-Laryngology

Vol. 69

Series Editor

W. Arnold Munich

Active Middle Ear Implants

Volume Editor

Klaus Böheim St. Pölten

25 figures, 4 in color, and 1 table, 2010

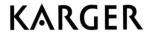

Basel · Freiburg · Paris · London · New York · Bangalore ·
Bangkok · Shanghai · Singapore · Tokyo · Sydney

Klaus Böheim
Department of Otorhinolaryngology
Head and Neck Surgery
Landesklinikum St. Pölten
Propst Führerstrasse 4
3100 St. Pölten (Austria)

Library of Congress Cataloging-in-Publication Data

Active middle ear implants / volume editor, Klaus Böheim.
      p. ; cm. -- (Advances in oto-rhino-laryngology, ISSN 0065-3071 ; v.
69)
  Includes bibliographical references and indexes.
  ISBN 978-3-8055-9470-7 (hard cover : alk. paper) -- ISBN 978-3-8055-9471-4
(e-ISBN)
  1. Hearing aids. 2. Implants, Artificial. 3. Middle ear--Surgery. I.
Böheim, Klaus. II. Series: Advances in oto-rhino-laryngology, v. 69.
0065-3071 ;
  [DNLM: 1. Ossicular Prosthesis. 2. Hearing Loss--surgery. 3. Ossicular
Replacement. W1 AD701 v.69 2010 / WV 230 A188 2010]
  RF305.A28 2010
  617.8'9--dc22
                                                2010017165

Bibliographic Indices. This publication is listed in bibliographic services, including Current Contents®.

© Copyright 2010 by S. Karger AG, P.O. Box, CH–4009 Basel (Switzerland)
www.karger.com
Printed in Switzerland on acid-free and non-aging paper (ISO 9706) by Reinhardt Druck, Basel
ISSN 0065–3071
ISBN 978–3–8055–9470–7
e-ISBN 978–3–8055–9471–4

Contents

Preface

I would like to sincerely thank the editor of *Advances in Oto-Rhino-Laryngology*, Prof. Wolfgang Arnold, for asking me to be guest editor for a book on active middle ear implants. It was a delightful undertaking for me to organize this anthology and to invite the authors who were selected from the many experts in the various topics of this broad field.

The publication of this book is very timely considering the recently expanded methods for coupling active middle ear implants to the middle ear – to the round window or in combination with passive middle ear prostheses. It is also an opportunity to review the currently marketed systems and to evaluate how they can be used to help hearing impaired patients. Over the past decade, we have witnessed a continuous evolution in the expansion of the patient selection criteria from purely sensorineural hearing losses to conductive and mixed hearing losses in difficult-to-treat ears.

This book begins with a fascinating and authentic history of active middle ear implants, written by one of the main pioneers in this field. In the following chapters, the currently marketed devices and their application are described. Technical improvements have resulted not only in better speech processing but also in fully implantable middle ear implants using electromagnetic stimulators. An additional development is the launch of a new, fully implantable device with a piezoelectric stimulator. Clinical experiences and results from a large group of patients, using the range of devices, are presented in this book.

I would like to extend my gratitude to all authors who prepared exceptionable manuscripts to share their experience. I am particularly thankful to Stefan-Marcel Pok for his hard work and long hours over many nights and weekends. His assistance contributed to the success of this publication.

Klaus Böheim, St. Pölten

Böheim K (ed): Active Middle Ear Implants.
Adv Otorhinolaryngol. Basel, Karger, 2010, vol 69, pp 1–13

The Vibrant Soundbridge: Design and Development

Geoffrey R. Ball

CTO Vibrant Med-El, Innsbruck, Austria

Abstract

This chapter is a condensed history of the design and development of the Vibrant Soundbridge that introduces and discusses the origins of the Floating Mass Transducer and the Vibrant Soundbridge and the design philosophy that led to the invention and realization of the system. The Vibrant Soundbridge has been worked on and studied by a large group of engineers, researchers, physicians and formal advisory boards whose combined efforts have led to approval for the system as it stands today. The system and operation as well as the possible future applications for middle ear implant technology are discussed. The author also thanks the many people that have contributed to the use and increasing adoption of the Vibrant Soundbridge to date.   Copyright © 2010 S. Karger AG, Basel

The goal to develop a superior electronic hearing system for the hearing impaired has had quite a history. Collins patented his first 'electronic hearing aid' in 1899 that featured a battery supply, amplifier and crude signal processing circuitry that drove a speaker (receiver) positioned in the ear canal. His device was crude; however, it possessed all the primary functional blocks of modern hearing aids in use today. Edison, arguably one of the greatest inventors of all time who suffered from severe hearing loss, also worked on improving the hearing aid and despite his successful work on microphones, electronics, amplifiers and batteries never commercialized a product and had to settle for founding the recording industry and many other feats. Work from the early 1900s through the 1980s was utilized to improve the packaging and function of components and then came the pioneering work of Villchur and Waldhaur that facilitated the introduction of active compression circuits that were the key breakthrough in hearing aid design [1, 2].

By recognizing that the hearing impaired had not only a loss in threshold levels, but also a decrease in dynamic range, the Villchur/Waldhaur technology was able to provide a compressed signal into the range that was most useful for the hearing impaired. For patients suffering from sensorineural hearing loss, this was a huge improvement. This technology was first introduced by ReSound Corporation. Today, almost all modern hearing systems utilize advanced signal compression. However, though a tremendous technical and clinical success, the introduction of advanced 'smart' hearing aid circuitry did not significantly alter hearing aid adoption patterns. Since the 1970s, the number of hearing aid 'owners' as a percentage of hearing impaired has varied between 21 and 23% [3]. This means that more than 75% of hearing loss sufferers that could and should benefit from amplification do not even own an instrument. A large portion of hearing aid 'owners' do not even utilize their hearing aid even once a year. The number of truly active hearing aid owners that use their devices four or more hours every day is 10% or less of the total hearing impaired population that could benefit.

The reason for rejection of hearing instruments by a clear majority of hearing loss sufferers is complicated and multifaceted. There is the stigma of hearing loss and wearing a hearing aid. There is the perceived lack of technology benefit; there are the many cases of unscrupulous hearing aid dispensing agents that have taken advantage by offering inferior technology at superior prices. There are the many patients that often have appropriate technology but have been unable to benefit due to inappropriate instrument fitting and/or programming of the unit to its full potential. Today, leading hearing aid companies are striving to increase adoption of amplification via educational awareness and marketing of their devices in the hope of improving adoption rates further than they have been historically. Although there have been significant improvements in total unit numbers for devices sold each year, frustratingly only incremental changes to the adoption rate as a percentage of total of sufferers have been made. A majority of cases that should be treated with amplification remain untreated despite technological improvement [3].

The field of direct-drive middle ear implant development has had quite a long history. The original theory behind middle ear development was that the primary Achilles' heel of acoustic hearing aids was that utilizing a speaker positioned near or about the ear canal introduced signal quality losses and the opportunity to imitate a feedback path. By introducing a device that was surgically implanted, patients could have the transducer positioned in much closer proximity to the ultimate target structure, the cochlea. Such a device could in theory deliver a superior signal without feedback and could offer improvements in cosmetics and ease of use for patients. Perhaps most importantly, for patients that have tried acoustic hearing aids and returned them who have utilized these devices for multiple years and desire an alternative, middle ear implants can offer an 'alternative' for long-term treatment, at least for some of them. There are hundreds of thousand of patients that can not actively wear acoustic hearing aids due to medical or anatomic reasons for which middle ear implants can and often do offer the best chance of hearing remediation. Acoustic hearing aids often offer limited benefit for many patients suffering form conductive or 'mixed' types of hearing deafness. Middle ear implants have been shown in many 'mixed' and conductive cases to have significant objective benefit and exceptional clinical utility.

With 80% or so of hearing impaired rejecting amplification, hearing loss is the single largest chronic sensory condition that typically remains untreated in medicine today. The need and demand for alternatives will only increase as the population grows and we will live longer, more productive lives. Proponents for alternative treatment options such as middle ear implants suggest that the many improvements and gains that can be achieved with this technology have been proven to benefit patients. They also argue that with a majority of sufferers with hearing loss remaining untreated there is a 'clear and obvious' need for alternatives for at least some patient categories. In contrast, the field of ophthalmology offers a host of alternative products and treatment options including prescription eyewear, contact lenses, corrective surgery and surgical options. The point is that for a majority of the visual impairments, more than one treatment option exists for most patients and there is a host of available products and service variants. The referral model and treatment pattern for vision impairments has been well tried and tested resulting in millions of surgical vision corrections each year. Certainly, a hearing implant or real technological or medical alternative to acoustic hearing aids can bring benefit to some portion of the population that forgoes treatment for their hearing loss. Interest in alternative treatments has brought many patients to audiology centers that may otherwise not have come and who ended up trying and adopting hearing aids. This is a good thing in my view.

More than USD 1 billion have been spent to date on the development of middle ear implants. The first serious well-funded attempts began with the early research work of Drs. Suzuki and Yanigihara in Japan, who were working in collaboration with the Rion hearing aid company. Though the early results were successful and quite promising, this piezo-electric device was never approved for commercialization and the device was applied in approximately 100 subjects in clinical investigations. A snapshot of other developments include Richards Medical (now Smith and Nephew) that worked on Jorgen Heide's middle ear electromagnetic total ossicular replacement prosthesis (TORP) device, the efforts of Perkins and Goode with the ReSound Earlens, the Implex TICA (totally implantable cochlea amplifier) and the work of many others including Maniglia, Hough, Spindel, Huettenbrink, etc. Though many of these devices and projects were significant technical achievements, in many events even stunning, for whatever reason, they have not been able to translate research and clinical achievements into commercial devices or achieve wide adoption in the field. On the one hand, this should not be a surprise as it is difficult to raise the capital required to develop an implant into form even for limited clinical trial use, and once this has been achieved to translate the research and clinical trials work into a commercially successful enterprise.

The result is that today the approved devices are the Envoy Esteem (formerly St. Croix Medical), the Carina (Otologics) and the Vibrant Soundbridge (Vibrant Med-

El). All three devices are approved and are in use within the EU and other countries. The Vibrant Soundbridge is unfortunately the only platform at the time of publishing that has been approved and is available for use in the US by the FDA since 2000. The other platforms are presently undergoing US clinical trials and we can hope to look forward to a future where several devices and designs are available. The good news is that although the number of devices that are in active use is small, the number of patients that are benefiting from these platforms continues to increase and interest is growing due to new indications and success with patients that need them.

Invention

Any good device requires a good invention. And good invention always has its share of good stories along the way. There have been many interesting moments in the development of the Vibrant Soundbridge and the invention of the FMT (Floating Mass Transducer). I can vividly recall the first time I thought about hearing implants. I was in Dr. Rodney Perkins' chair as a patient, and we were finishing the examination and reviewing my test results and so I asked him 'What about surgery, is there anything that you can do to fix me up?' 'No, not that would help your loss' he replied. And so I said 'What about a hearing implant, an implanted device like one of those cochlear implants.' And he replied 'No, those won't help you but we are working on something, so in a couple years it could be a possibility.' I could not have envisioned that only a few short years later I would be employed by his colleague Dr. Richard Goode and working on that very project. I could have had no idea that hearing implants and the sciences surrounding this field would become my life's work.

Noninventors often seem to think that the process of invention involves and leads to a 'Eureka!' moment. A moment where the light bulb of the brain fires big and the idea presents itself and one thinks 'by Jove I've got it!' Well for the FMT this was not the way that it happened. There was no true 'Eureka!' moment. It was a process that took many years. First, I had to understand the problem, study the ear, carry out countless dissections and engage in basic research studies. We had to perform live human studies to identify the vibrational patterns and use cadavers to try different ideas and concepts. Along the way, I had to adapt and perfect several test methods and measurement devices for basic and applied research, and then eventually develop bench testing and ultimately manufacturing tests for the incredibly small and sensitive devices required for direct drive of the middle ear. I had to design and build, often by hand in my father's workshop late at night, new transducers. Hundreds of variants were tried and all failed for one reason or the other. All had one or more shortcomings or did not work at all.

In graduate school at USC, I had taken a class in the rather obscure field of linear programming. I tried to set up the problem of middle ear implants into a linear programming model to maximize the variants that needed to be maximized (output,

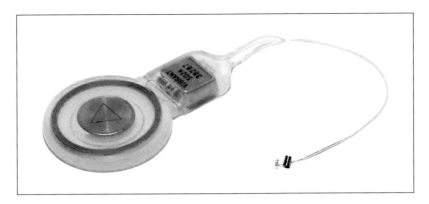

Fig. 2. Vibrating ossicular prosthesis.

supplies power to the system. The AP sends an amplitude modulated signal across the skin to the receiver coil of the VORP. The AP is held in position postauricularly on the outside of the head during normal use by magnetic attraction.

The VORP is implanted during the surgical procedure and consists of three functional components. These units are:

(a) Implanted receiver unit: the implanted receiver unit receives the electromagnetic signal from the external amplification system. A demodulator circuit filters the modulated signal to the appropriate drive signal for the FMT.

(b) Conductor link: the conductor link functions as the electrical conduit that connects the FMT to the implanted receiver unit.

(c) Floating mass transducer: the FMT drives a vibratory structure of an ear.

The important components of the VORP include the receiver coil; a polymide-coated gold wire that is inductively matched to the telemetry coil of the AP. The magnet attachment assembly, located in the center of the receiver coil, functions as the attachment magnet that holds the AP in its proper external position.

An additional component of the VORP is the demodulation electronic package which contains an array of passive electronic components (resistors, capacitors and diodes) assembled on a ceramic substrate. The demodulation electronics package provides three functions: (1) it demodulates the drive signal transmitted to the VORP by the AP, (2) it protects the transducer from any potential interference sources, and (3) it limits the output of the FMT to obviate any opportunity for overstimulation.

Vibrant Soundbridge Theory of Operation

When an acoustic signal reaches the microphone (or microphones) of the AP, it is converted into an electronic signal. This signal is then processed by the signal-processing electronics and the resultant signal is then amplified and modulated into the appropriate drive signal, which is then transmitted across the skin to the VORP. The receiver coil of the VORP picks up the modulated signal broadcasted by the AP and sends it to the demodulation electronics package where the signal is demodulated and sent down the conductor link to the FMT. The FMT then mechanically vibrates the ossicular chain with amplified motion, ultimately stimulating the fluid of the inner ear. The user then experiences amplified sound.

Rather than using acoustic sound as the drive force, the Vibrant Soundbridge delivers mechanical energy to the ossicular chain. In the partially implantable Soundbridge, the microphone of the externally worn AP picks up sound. The AP is held in position under a patient's hair by magnetic attraction. The AP's microphone picks up sound (note: the latest AP has two microphones) and the resultant electronic signal is amplified and sent to the internally located receiver portion of the VORP. The signal is passed down the conductor link to the FMT located on the most distal portion of the VORP. The FMT then delivers mechanical motion to the ear.

To date, several thousands of subjects have been implanted with the Vibrant Soundbridge for sensorineural, conductive and mixed hearing loss. The benefits of the direct-drive devices for the majority of patients have been reported in over 50 publications to date. The AP has been continuously upgraded to take advantage of improvements in signal processing technology and to accommodate other design changes that have resulted in improved patient performance.

The advantage of a system that has a minimal effect on patient's residual hearing cannot be overstated. For any medical technology, no matter how well tested in advance, a thorough clinical study will reveal the true strengths and weaknesses of a device's design. Studies on the Vibrant Soundbridge reveal a device that is appropriate for the prescribed indication range for sensori-neural, mixed and conductive hearing loss. The strengths, merits and areas for future improvement for the Vibrant Soundbridge have been illustrated well in many peer-reviewed publications and clinical trial reports that describe the function, performance and limits of the Vibrant Soundbridge. These will be continually augmented and updated and as I write this (October, 2009) we have just got back the first reports for the latest Amadé AP which were much better than we anticipated including much higher gain in the entire audiofrequency range (including the low frequencies) and impressive speech improvements in quiet and in noise settings. The ability for hearing improvement from improved signal processing is key to any hearing system in my view and is a key advantage of the present version of the Vibrant Soundbridge.

The Future

Since 1999, all the basic technology has existed for us to construct a totally implantable system. In my view, the main stumbling block has always been and will continue to be the battery. Rechargeable batteries have been long overdue for a major breakthrough that affords a truly significant increase in cell capacity.

TI (totally implantable) devices have arrived on the scene and are taking their first steps in the field as commercial products. I believe that a TI device really has to be more or less 'perfect' because the signal processing and upgrades cannot be readily changed as we can do with externally worn APs. As a hearing impaired person, I struggle with the question as to how often does the average person truly need a TI? I really don't want to hear or need to hear acoustic sound when I am underwater or swimming laps. And when showering for a few minutes, well yes, I cannot wear an AP in the shower either, but I think this is a minor inconvenience, not a strong rational for a TI. I do, however, believe that the TI will become a good option one day in the future, especially once the batteries have improved and the devices can be made even smaller than they are now and offer specific human-factor advantages and cosmetics for patients that do not have enough hair. I also think that in the future they could be particularly well suited for children and exceptionally for athletic individuals. However, there are also benefits for transcutaneous partially implanted systems that are undeniable and so I reckon there will be a need for both in the foreseeable future. The main benefit for TI design at present appears to be and do with cosmetic and perceptual issues. So far, increased performance from the TI configuration above partially implantable systems has not been proven. However, I am quite certain that there is a lot more to the TI riddle that we need to and will come to understand better. What design components do we maximize, what do we need to minimize and what are the right trade-offs from a design perspective? What are the right inputs and deliverables? What human factors improvements can be made and what are the performance benefits? It is my view that a TI device should ideally work at least as well and preferably better than a transcutaneous system in terms of gain and output and speech improvement scores. My guess would be that the TI concept will be most relevant and perhaps most important for cochlear implant users, but we shall see how the topic develops.

At present, many new implant designs are being worked on and are speeding down the development pipeline. There is much to be excited about! My personal view is that I now think that the 'Holy Grail' for hearing devices may not be one specific device or one specific design permutation, but rather the ability to support and deliver a complete family of devices for the treatment of differing hearing loss types and degrees. In other words, instead of one perfect 'stand alone' system, perfection is likely to rather be in the arrival of a plurality of implant designs and configurations with different stimulation types, or a combination of operational modes that, when taken together, can remediate the majority of hearing loss cases in need of alternative treatment with an arsenal of approaches that can be deployed in the surgical theater.

Conclusion

We believe that the device that is now approved for use today is the realization and culmination of several disciplines working together towards a common goal, i.e. the development of a surgical treatment for hearing loss. This arena offers hope and help for many hearing-impaired patients and for many expanded indications. As research in this area continues, we expect to see new developments that continue to improve direct-drive technology and expand the ability of the technology to address additional hearing loss categories.

Acknowledgements

There is no letter 'I' in the word 'team'. Dr. Goode approved the appropriate rights to the FMT to be assigned to me by applying to the 'Technology Transfer Office' for transfer of my inventions. I also need to extend Ugo Fisch unending gratitude for his help with the input into the basic design concept and in particular work on the lead, size and developmental work on the surgical method for the VORP and for his participation in the original SAB meetings. In addition to Ugo Fisch as the PI of the EU VSB clinical trial, key participants include Cor Cremers, Thomas Lenarz, Benno Weber, Gregorio Babighian, Alain Uziel, David Proops, Alec F. O'Connor, Robert Charchon, Jan Helms and Bernard Fraysse. Anders Tjellstrom published the results of our first 'Acute Trial of the Vibrant Soundbridge' in 1997 and was the first to publish the observation that the VSB could 'also be used to treat conductive hearing loss'. The first patient was implanted by Ugo Fisch in 1996. The first known use of the Vibrant Soundbridge to clinically treat conductive and mixed loss was by Thibaud DuMon in France, Vittorio Colletti pioneered the use of the FMT in alternative locations on the RW beginning in 2005. Key breakthrough! There were so many others with so many 'firsts' that helped us along the way that to come up with a complete list without leaving someone off that should be on it would be quite an impossible task!

In the USA, Dr. Hough was the 'Principal Investigator' for the Vibrant Soundbridge clinical trials and he and his team including Dr. Stan Baker, Dr. Dormer and Dr. Gan helped tremendously with the development of our original surgical development along with the help from all their team members. The invaluable work of other surgeons that participated in the SAB and clinical trials included (but are not limited to) Charlie Luetje, Derald Brackman, Thomas Balkany, Jennifer Maw, David Kelsall, Douglas Backous, Richard Miyamoto, Simon Parisier and Alexander Arts. There were also many USA audiologists that helped with our clinical trial work including Deborah Arthur, Christine Menapace, Pamela Mathews, Darcy Benson, Theresa Clarke, Charles Berlin and many more. The attachment clip project was completed by Chris Julian with the help of the SAB input. The implant attachment magnet concept for the VORP we licensed from the University of Oklahoma, the original size for the FMT (same as it is today) was again arrived at with Ugo Fisch and others and in T-bone studies conducted by me and Stan Baker. The surgery was developed again with the SAB members in the EU and USA and the original implant telemetry scheme was based on the work that Erwin and Ingeborg Hochmair used for cochlear implants. Hans Camenzind was my original 'Angel' investor, followed by B.J. Cassin, Peter McNerney and Karen Bozie. Ron Antipa helped me with the original business plans and to arrange the funding for Symphonix and to him I am eternally grateful.

On the Symphonix design team, we had Bob Katz, Craig Mar, Dan Wallace, Chris Julian, Tim Dietz, Eric Jaeger, Duane Tumlinson and Frank Fellenz on the implant side. On the AP development side, there was Bruce Arthur, Jim Culp, John Salsbury, Steve Trebotich, Wyn Robertson and several other engineers. Manufacturing the tiny FMTs was developed by Pat Rimroth, Ahn Troung and Sue Clarke. Many of these people are listed on the patents where they had made appropriate contributions resulting in issued claims. Bruce Maxfield and I developed the original detailed mathematics that describe how FMTs work. Special thanks to Peter Hertzman, Alf Merriweather, Beth Anne McDonald, Jeff Rydin, Mike Arendt, the Symphonix sales and clinical support staff, and the many other key support personnel from Symphonix times. Today, the VSB is supported by our R&D staff including Peter Lampbacher, Marcus Shmidt, Klaus Holzer, Ali Mayr, Markus Nagl, Michael Santek, Klaus Triendl, Bernd Gerhardter and many others on the RA, QA and clinical sides and of course Ingeborg Hochmair as CEO. She saved the Vibrant Soundbridge and has been the greatest! I would also like to thank all the people that helped on the 'save the Vibrant Soundbridge project' by moving the operating assets from San Jose, Calif. to our new home in Austria. Especially Alexander Mayr, Linda Ferner, Martin Kerber, Walter Fimml, Klaus Holzer and the Med-El transfer team.

Then of course there are the many others that have helped me out personally including Joe Roberson, Klaus Boeheim, Wolfgang Baumgartner, Alex Huber, Norbert Dillier, Timothy Wild, Thomas Lenarz, Jon Spindel, Michel Beliaff, Bill Perry, Joachim Mueller and Harry Robbins. Special thanks also go to Jan Helms for his willingness to spend extra time with me over the years. Invaluable all! For the many researchers that have contributed original work I thank you! I think there are too many to list again and I applaud the many people that have earned higher academic PhDs and other degrees for 'original work' for the Vibrant Soundbridge, FMT and related topics. Thanks to the entire Japanese team at Ehime for working with me all these years! Again, thanks to Dr. Goode, who imprinted his view of hearing and the world of all things otology, engineering, medical, philosophical, design and invention wise upon me and my paltry inferior brain comparatively. He was a great teacher and mentor, and I thank him so much for believing in and taking a chance on me. And sorry for the days when the Goode maxim 'When the surf is good the lab ain't doing what it should!' was sometimes correct. Be assured those were epic days!

We always say we are treating hearing loss, we are doing so much more for so many, we are really giving people new and better lives and enjoyment of the world of sound and helping to reduce hearing loss as a barrier to communication with others.

As for me. I'm not yet finished. I assure you.

References

1 Villchur E: Signal processing to improve speech intelligibility in perceptive deafness. J Acoust Soc Am 1973;53:1646–1657.
2 Villchur E: Simulation of the effect of recruitment on loudness relationships in speech (demonstration disk bound in with article). J Acoust Soc Am 1974; 56:1601–1611.
3 Kochkin S: Hearing Review – July 2005. MarkeTrak VII: Hearing Loss Population Tops 31 Million (available online at www.hearingreview.com).
4 Goode RL, Ball G, Nishihara S, Nakamura K: Laser Doppler vibrometer (LDV) – a new clinical tool for the otologist. Am J Otol 1996;17:813–822.

Geoffrey R. Ball
CTO Vibrant Med-El
Fürstenweg 77
AT–6020 Innsbruck (Austria)
Tel. +43 0 512 28 88 89 251, Fax +43 0 512 28 88 89 299, E-Mail geoff.ball@medel.com

Böheim K (ed): Active Middle Ear Implants.
Adv Otorhinolaryngol. Basel, Karger, 2010, vol 69, pp 14–19

Cost-Effectiveness of Implantable Middle Ear Hearing Devices

Ad Snik · Veronique Verhaegen · Jef Mulder · Cor Cremers

Department of Otorhinolaryngology, Radboud University Nijmegen Medical Center, Nijmegen,
The Netherlands

Abstract

Objective: To assess the relation between cost and effectiveness of implantable middle ear hearing devices in patients with pure sensorineural hearing loss. **Design:** Literature review. **Results:** Four studies were identified that described the effect of middle ear implantation on quality of life in groups of at least 20 patients. Several different quality of life questionnaires were used. **Conclusions:** Our review demonstrated that middle ear implantation is a cost-effective health care intervention in patients with sensorineural hearing loss who suffered an additional therapy-resistant chronic external otitis.

Middle ear implantation is a relatively new treatment for patients with sensorineural hearing loss who do not benefit from conventional hearing aid fitting. Today's middle ear hearing aids are still semi-implantable devices. They comprise an audioprocessor with microphone, electronics and FM transmitter, which is worn externally. The audioprocessor is in (magnetic) contact with an implanted receiver unit, placed just below the skin in the mastoid region [1]. This receiver is connected to the output transducer that is coupled to one of the middle ear ossicles.

Recently, middle ear implants have been applied to patients with conductive or mixed hearing loss. The transducer is coupled directly to the cochlea via one of the cochlear windows [2].

In contrast to a conventional hearing aid, the application of a middle ear implant involves surgery and much higher financial costs. These features have led to health-economic questions regarding treatment effectiveness in relation to the cost.

Let us first consider effectiveness. To assess the effect of a medical intervention on a patient's feeling of well-being, questionnaires are often administered. One option is the use of generic health-related quality of life (HR-QoL) questionnaires, such as the

Short Form 36 (SF-36) [3, 4], the EuroQol [5] or the Health Utility Index [6]. In principle, these HR-QoL questionnaires are not disease-specific and can therefore be applied across the borders of a specific disability. The main outcome of most generic HR-QoL questionnaires is one single measure called utility. It ranges between 1 (perfectly happy) and 0 (death). The change in utility owing to a specific intervention is called the utility gain and it is used to determine the quality-adjusted life-years or QALYs. A QALY is the utility gain in a group of patients multiplied by the life expectancy after the intervention [7, 8]. The second option is to use hearing handicap-specific QoL questionnaires.

Several studies that used generic HR-QoL questionnaire scores showed only small changes in utility gain after conventional hearing aid fitting [9]. This is in direct contrast with handicap-specific questionnaires that mostly demonstrated significant improvements [10]. It has been concluded that most generic HR-QoL questionnaires are not sensitive to problems associated with audition and communication [9, 11]. Furthermore, when different HR-QoL questionnaires were used in parallel to assess the benefit of hearing interventions, wide interquestionnaire variability was found [11, 12]. Therefore, handicap-specific questionnaires have been introduced to measure QoL after hearing interventions and they have become very popular. Examples are the Glasgow Benefit Inventory [13], the Nijmegen Cochlear Implant Questionnaire [14, 15] and the International Outcome Inventory for hearing aid provision [16]. These questionnaires have well-described structures and have been validated; however, they do not provide utility scores. Let us take a closer look at these questionnaires.

The Glasgow Benefit Inventory (GBI): The GBI is a HR-QoL questionnaire that was specially developed to measure outcomes of otorhinolaryngological interventions; it is a retrospective standardized questionnaire that examines the impact of the treatment on the health status of the patient [13]. Scores can range from –100 (profound deterioration) to +100 (excellent improvement). Twelve of the 18 questions are about general health, 3 questions concern social functioning and 3 concern physical health. The GBI has been used successfully to evaluate the bone-anchored hearing aid [14] and cochlear implants [15].

The Nijmegen Cochlear Implant Questionnaire (NCIQ): The NCIQ is an HR-QoL questionnaire that was specially developed to assess longitudinal health status after cochlear implantation [16, 17]. It addresses three functional domains: physical (communication related), social and psychological functioning. Each subdomain contains at least 10 items. The overall scores per subdomain range from 0 (very poor) to 100 (optimal).

The three domains showed acceptable consistency statistics, test-retest coefficients and responsiveness indexes [16, 17]. In a long-term follow-up study on adults with cochlear implants, the NCIQ scores were fairly consistent over time [18]. Nowadays, the NCIQ is being widely used [18–22]. It has been used for example to compare quality of life between cochlear implant users and hearing aid users with severe hearing loss [18, 22].

The International Outcome Inventory for Hearing Aids (IOI-HA): This seven-item, self-report survey has been translated into more than 20 languages [23]. Each of the seven items targets a different field, namely daily use, benefit, residual activity limitation, satisfaction, residual participation restriction, impact on others and quality of life. Scores range from 1 (poor) to 5 (optimal). The psychometric properties have been studied extensively and norms have been established from large groups of conventional hearing aid users [23].

Cost-Utility Ratio of Hearing Intervention

The direct cost of treatment can be divided into the phases of selection, implantation and rehabilitation [7, 8, 24]. To calculate the cost-per-QALY of middle ear implantation, we need to know the direct cost and utility gain. However, owing to the variation in utility scores across generic HR-QoL questionnaires, as referred to above, such calculations are not straightforward. Let us look at the cost-per-QALY determination of conventional hearing aid fitting according to Grutters et al. [12]. They used four different generic HR-QoL questionnaires in parallel to assess a group of 315 patients who had been fitted with hearing aids for the first time. Utility gain values obtained with the four questionnaires differed by a factor of 40 and, as a consequence, the calculated cost-per-QALY also differed by this unacceptable range of 40. Thus, the cost-per-QALY seems to primarily depend on the generic HR-QoL questionnaire used and not on the effectiveness of the intervention or its cost. Therefore, any health-economic evaluation of hearing interventions based on the cost-per-QALY concept can be questioned.

Handicap-specific QoL might form an alternative way to assess cost utility. As cochlear implantation in postlingually deaf adults has an acceptable cost-utility ratio [7, 8, 25], the effectiveness of a new type of implantation might be determined by comparing the outcomes of handicap-specific QoL questionnaires after the new treatment to those of cochlear implantation. Next, the cost of the new intervention must be calculated and compared to that of cochlear implantation. Based on the relative effectiveness and the relative cost, it can be concluded whether or not the new treatment is more or less cost-effective than cochlear implantation [26].

Quality of Life and Middle Ear Implantation: A Review of the Literature

QoL in relation to middle ear implantation was studied in a substantially large group of patients (n ≥ 20) in four papers [26–29]. Sterkers et al. [27] published the results of a French multicenter trial on patients with pure sensorineural hearing loss, implanted with the Vibrant Soundbridge middle ear hearing device (Med-El, Innsbruck, Austria). They used the inclusion criteria advocated by the manufacturer. Recently, long-term data have been published on the same group [28]. To evaluate patient benefit, the

Table 1. Mean GBI data from 3 different studies: total score and mean scores per subdomain are presented

	Study			
	Snik et al. [26]	Sterkers et al. [27]	Mosnier et al. [28]	Schmuziger et al. [29]
Number of patients	17	57	62	20
GBI score				
Total	32.9	15.4	17.8	14.7
General score	41.5	20.0	22.8	22.1
Physical health	15.7	0.0	1.7	−5.0
Social interaction	17.6	11.5	14.1	5.0

GBI was used. In 57 patients, the mean overall improvement was 15 points (on a scale from −100 to +100) in the initial study and 18 points in the long-term study [27, 28, respectively]. Table 1 presents the mean scores on each of the three GBI subscales.

Schmuziger et al. [29] published their retrospective data on a group of 20 Vibrant Soundbridge users with pure sensorineural hearing loss. They also employed the inclusion criteria advocated by Med-El. The GBI and the IOI-HA were applied to obtain data. Overall improvement on the GBI was 15 points (table 1), while the IOI-HA showed an overall postintervention score of 3.7 (on a scale from 1 to 5). For reference purposes, the authors compared their results to the norm data reported by Cox et al. [23]. After conventional hearing aid fitting, the mean norm score in the latter study was 3.6, which was almost the same as the IOI-HA score from the middle ear implant users.

Snik et al. [26] presented the results of a prospective quality of life study on 21 patients with sensorineural hearing loss who received a middle ear implant. The devices comprised either the Vibrant Soundbridge or the Otologics MET (Otologics Company, Boulder, Colo., USA). Treatment cost was determined based on the direct cost of implantation, rehabilitation and 1 year of aftercare. The total cost was EUR 14,354 per middle ear implant, irrespective of the type. To assess effectiveness, the patients filled out the generic SF-36 and NCIQ before and at 6 and 12 months after implantation [26]. The GBI was filled out once, between 6 and 12 months after implantation. In contrast with the other three papers, the patients described by Snik et al. [26] were all suffering from chronic, therapy-resistant external otitis. The SF-36 outcome showed only minimal improvement after the intervention. In agreement with Brazier et al. [4], the mean utility gain on the SF-36 was 0.01 (on a scale from 0 to 1). This small improvement in SF-36 utility is explained by the statement in the Introduction section that most generic HR-QoL questionnaires are too insensitive to hearing problems. Based on this utility gain, the cost-per-QALY was high: it exceeded EUR 70,000. In contrast, all three domains of the NCIQ showed substantial improvement in the scores after middle ear implantation ($p \leq 0.01$), while the mean GBI score was 33 points, which indicated a highly significant improvement ($p < 0.001$).

Next, Snik et al. [26] compared the middle ear implantation NCIQ subscale scores to those obtained in their previous cochlear implant study on postlingually deaf adults [16, 17]. Analyses showed that cochlear implantation was 1.5–2.5 times more effective than middle ear implantation, whereas middle ear implantation was 3.3 times cheaper than cochlear implantation. These findings suggest that middle ear implantation is more cost-effective than cochlear implantation.

The GBI score in the study by Snik et al. [26] was considerably higher than that reported in the other studies (table 1). This might have been due to their inclusion criterion of external otitis. Such patients cannot tolerate an ear mould, or they can only tolerate the occlusion for a few hours per day. A middle ear implant enabled these patients to hear again without any pain or itching in the ears. Table 1 shows that this group of patients had higher GBI scores throughout. The most profound difference was seen in the physical health domain.

As stated above, all the patients studied by Snik et al. [26] had comorbid external otitis in contrast with Sterkers et al. [27] and Schmuziger et al. [29], whose patients comprised dissatisfied conventional hearing aid users alone. The relatively low GBI scores reported by Sterkers et al. [27], Mosnier et al. [28] and Schmuziger et al. [29] indicate limited benefit. This conclusion is in agreement with the post-intervention IOI-HA scores presented by Schmuziger et al. [29]. Their IOI-HA scores showed that middle ear implants did not have a surplus value compared to conventional hearing aids.

In conclusion, middle ear implantation seemed to be cost-effective in patients with sensorineural hearing loss and with comorbid chronic external otitis. Our literature review suggested that this conclusion may not apply to patients with pure sensorineural hearing loss who dislike conventional air-conduction devices for whatever reason and are searching for an alternative.

References

1 Miller DA, Fredrickson JM: Implantable hearing aids; in Valente M, Hosford-Dunn H, Roeser RJ (eds): Audiology: Treatment. New York, Thieme Medical Publishers, 2000, pp 489–510.

2 Colletti V, Soli SD, Carner M, Colletti L: Treatment of mixed hearing losses via implantation of a vibratory transducer on the round window. Int J Audiol 2006;45:600–608.

3 Ware JE, Sherbourne CD: The MOS 36-item short-form health survey (SF-36): conceptual framework and item selection. Med Care 1992;30:473–483.

4 Brazier J, Roberts J, Deverill M: The estimation of a preference-based measure of health from the SF-36. J Health Econ 2002;21:271–292.

5 The EuroQol Group: EuroQol – a new facility for the measurement of health-related quality of life. Health Policy 1990;16:199–208.

6 Feeny D, Furlong W, Torrance GW, Goldsmith CH, Zhu Z, DePauw S, Denton M, Boyle M: Multi-attribute and single-attribute utility functions for the health utilities index mark 3 system. Med Care 2002;40:113–128.

7 UKCISG (UK Cochlear Implant Study Group). Criteria of candidacy for unilateral cochlear implantation in postlingually deafened adults. II. Cost-effectiveness analysis. Ear Hear 2004;25:336–360.

8 Palmer CS, Niparko JK, Wyatt JR, Rothman R, De Lissovoy G: A prospective study of the cost-utility of the multichannel cochlear implant. Arch Otolaryngol Head Neck Surg 1999;125:1221–1218.

9 Bess FH: The role of generic health-related quality of life measures in establishing audiological rehabilitation outcomes. Ear Hear 2000;21:74S–79S.

10 Chisolm TH, Johnson CE, Danhauer JL, Potz LJP, Abrams HB, Lesner S, McCarthy PA, Newman CW: A systematic review of health-related quality of life and hearing aids: final report of the American Academy task force on the health-related quality of life benefits of amplification in adults. J Am Acad Audiol 2007;18:151–183.

11 Barton GR, Bankart J, Davis AC, Summerfield QA: Comparing utility scores before and after hearing aid provision: results to the EQ-5D, HUI3 and SF-6D. Appl Health Econ Health Policy 2004;3:103–105.

12 Grutters JPC, Joore MA, van der Horst F, Dreschler WA, Anteunis LJC: Choosing between measures: comparison of EQ-5D, HUI2, HUI3 in persons with hearing complaints. Qual Life Res 2007;16: 1439–1449.

13 Robinson K, Gatehouse S, Browning GC: Measuring benefit from otorhinolaryngological surgery and therapy. Ann Otol Rhino Laryngol 1996;105: 415–422.

14 Krabbe PFM, Hinderink JB, Van den Broek P: The effect of cochlear implant use in postlingually deaf adults. Int J Technol Assess Health Care 2000;16: 864–873.

15 Snik AFM, Mylanus EAM, Proops DW, Wolfaardt JF, Hodgetts WE, Somers T, Niparko JK, Wazen JJ, Sterkers O, Cremers CW, Tjellström A: Consensus statements on the BAHA system: where do we stand at present? Ann Otol Rhinol Laryngol Suppl 2005; 195:2–12.

16 UKCISG (UK Cochlear Implant Study Group). Criteria of candidacy for unilateral cochlear implantation in postlingually deafened adults I: Theory and measures of effectiveness. Ear Hear 2004;25:310–335.

17 Hinderink JB, Krabbe PFM, Van den Broek P: Development and application of a health related quality of life instrument for adults with cochlear implants: the Nijmegen Cochlear Implant Questionnaire. Otolaryngol Head Neck Surg 2000;123: 756–765.

18 Damen GW, Beynon AJ, Krabbe PF, Mulder JJ, Mylanus EA: Cochlear implantation and quality of life in postlingually deaf adults: long-term follow-up. Otolaryngol Head Neck Surg 2007;136:597–604.

19 Klop WM, Boermans PP, Ferrier MB, van den Hout WB, Stiggelbout AM, Frijns JH: Clinical relevance of quality of life outcome in cochlear implantation in postlingually deafened adults. Otol Neurotol 2008:29;615–621.

20 Baumgartner WD, Jappel A, Morera C, Gstöttner W, Müller J, Kiefer J, Van De Heyning P, Anderson I, Nielsen SB: Outcomes in adults implanted with the FLEX soft electrode. Acta Otolaryngol 2007; 127:579–586.

21 Hirschfelder A, Gräbel S, Olze H: The impact of cochlear implantation on quality of life: the role of audiologic performance and variables. Otolaryngol Head Neck Surg 2008;138:357–362

22 Cohen SM, Labadie RF, Dietrich MS, Haynes DS: Quality of life in hearing-impaired adults: the role of cochlear implants and hearing aids. Otolaryngol Head Neck Surg 2004;131:413–422.

23 Cox RM, Alexander GC, Beyer CM: Norms for the International Outcome Inventory for Hearing Aids. J Am Acad Audiol 2003;14:403–413.

24 Severens JL, Bokx JPL, Van den Broek P: Cost analysis of cochlear implants in deaf children in the Netherlands. Am J Otol 1997;18:714–718.

25 Cheng AK, Niparko JK: Cost-utility of cochlear implant in adults: a meta-analysis. Arch Otolaryngol Head Neck Surg 1999;125:1214–1218.

26 Snik AF, van Duijnhoven NT, Mylanus EA, Cremers CW: Estimated cost-effectiveness of active middle-ear implantation in hearing-impaired patients with severe external otitis. Arch Otolaryngol Head Neck Surg 2006;132:1210–1215.

27 Sterkers O, Boucarra D, Labassi S, Bebear J-P, Dubreuil C, Frachet B, Fraysse B, Lavieille J-P, Magnan J, Martin C, Truy E, Uziel A, Vaneecloo FM: A middle ear implant, the Symphonix Vibrant Soundbridge: retrospective study of the first 125 patients implanted in France. Otol Neurotol 2003;24:427–436.

28 Mosnier I, Sterkers O, Bouccara D, Labassi S, Bebear JP, Bordure P, Dubreuil C, Dumon T, Frachet B, Fraysse B, Lavieille JP, Magnan J, Martin C, Meyer B, Mondain M, Portmann D, Robier A, Schmerber S, Thomassin JM, Truy E, Uziel A, Vaneecloo FM, Vincent C, Ferrary E: Benefit of the Vibrant Soundbridge device in patients implanted for 5 to 8 years. Ear Hear 2008;29:281–284.

29 Schmuziger N, Schimmann F, àWengen D, Patscheke J, Probst R: Long-term assessment after implantation of the Vibrant Soundbridge device. Otol Neurotol 2006;27:183–188.

A. Snik
ENT Department – 377, Radboud University Nijmegen Medical Centre
PO Box 9101
NL–6500 HB Nijmegen (The Netherlands)
Tel. +31 243 614 927, E-Mail a.snik@kno.umcn.nl

Böheim K (ed): Active Middle Ear Implants.
Adv Otorhinolaryngol. Basel, Karger, 2010, vol 69, pp 20–26

Indications and Candidacy for Active Middle Ear Implants

F. Wagner · I. Todt · J. Wagner · A. Ernst

Department of Otolaryngology, ukb, Hospital of the University of Berlin (Charité Medical School), Berlin, Germany

Abstract

Currently, there are two active middle ear implants available commercially: the Vibrant Soundbridge system and the Carina system. A third active middle ear implant, the Esteem, is under clinical evaluation. All devices are indicated for patients with moderate-to-severe hearing loss. Because active middle ear implants are directly coupled to middle ear structures, many of the problems that patients with conventional hearing aids report, such as acoustic feedback, occlusion, and irritation of the outer ear canal, are avoided. In addition, AMEI patients perform well in background noise. However, indications for AMEIs are selective and candidates should be carefully evaluated before surgery. Before considering an AMEI, patients should be provided with conventional hearing aids. Only when benefit is insufficient and audiological selection criteria are met is further candidacy evaluation indicated. Since Colletti described coupling the Vibrant Soundbridge directly onto the round window membrane in 2006, the indications for the Vibrant Soundbridge have expanded and the VSB is implanted in patients with conductive and mixed hearing losses. Patients have often undergone middle ear surgery before. Especially mixed hearing loss cases with 30–60 dB HL sensorineural hearing impairment and 30–40 dB HL air-bone gaps may be helped by this new application.

Copyright © 2010 S. Karger AG, Basel

Active middle ear implants (AMEIs) have been implanted for more than 10 years. Today's commercially available AMEIs are manufactured by MED-EL, Innsbruck, Austria (the Vibrant Soundbridge, VSB [1–4]) and by Otologics LLC, Boulder, Colo., USA (the Carina [2, 5, 6]). The Esteem AMEI from Envoy Medical Corporation, Minneapolis, Minn., USA, has the CE mark as all the other systems above. There have been other systems that were not developed into commercial products and have not been approved [7–12].

The indication for AMEIs is primarily based on audiological criteria. AMEIs are indicated for patients with moderate-to-severe sensorineural hearing loss (SNHL), who have not undergone middle ear surgery before and have been unsuccessfully treated delivers energy to the cochlea with the second lead wire. Because tympanic membrane movement is connected to the implant, no microphone is necessary. Patient access to the implant is provided by a remote control device. An additional operation, after about 4 years, is needed to replace the internal battery. Because the implant connects to the ossicles and senses tympanic membrane movement, the candidate should not have had previous middle ear surgery, and unobstructed tympanic membrane and ossicular chain movement is required.

Conclusions

Active middle ear implants have provided an alternative to conventional hearing aids for hearing-impaired patients over the past decade. They are an option for patients who cannot be sufficiently rehabilitated with conventional hearing aids or surgical techniques such as tympanoplasty.

The number of candidates for AMEIs is limited and patients should be selected carefully. Patients who are candidates are usually not satisfied with their hearing aids. The alternative treatment, the AMEI, usually results in good patient satisfaction. The new approach for the VSB provides new possibilities for patients with mixed hearing loss and previous middle ear surgeries. Especially for hearing losses with a 30- to 60-dB HL sensorineural component and a 30- to 40-dB HL conductive hearing loss, it is now possible to offer a reliable treatment to patients who previously had no alternative to conventional hearing aids.

References

1 Gan RZ, Wood MW, Ball GR, Dietz TG, Dormer KJ: Implantable hearing device performance measured by laser Doppler interferometry. Ear Nose Throat J 1997;76:297–299, 302, 305–309.
2 Snik A, Noten J, Cremers C: Gain and maximum output of two electromagnetic middle ear implants: are real ear measurements helpful? J Am Acad Audiol 2004;15:pp 249–257.
3 Snik AF, Cremers CW: Vibrant semi-implantable hearing device with digital sound processing: effective gain and speech perception. Arch Otolaryngol Head Neck Surg 2001;127:1433–1437.
4 Sterkers O, Boucarra D, Labassi S, Bebear JP, Dubreuil C, Frachet B, Fraysse B, Lavieille JP, Magnan J, Martin C, Truy E, Uziel A, Vaneecloo FM: A middle ear implant, the Symphonix Vibrant Soundbridge: retrospective study of the first 125 patients implanted in France. Otol Neurotol 2003;24:427–436.
5 Jenkins HA, Niparko JK, Slattery WH, Neely JG, Fredrickson JM: Otologics Middle Ear Transducer Ossicular Stimulator: performance results with varying degrees of sensorineural hearing loss. Acta Otolaryngol 2004;124:391–394.
6 Kasic JF, Fredrickson JM: The Otologics MET ossicular stimulator. Otolaryngol Clin North Am 2001;34:501–513.
7 Perkins R: Earlens tympanic contact transducer: a new method of sound transduction to the human ear. Otolaryngol Head Neck Surg 1996;114:720–728.
8 Yanagihara N, Aritomo H, Yamanaka E, Gyo K: Implantable hearing aid: report of the first human applications. Arch Otolaryngol Head Neck Surg 1987;113:869–872.

9 Maniglia AJ, Ko WH, Rosenbaum M, Zhu WL, Werning J, Belser R, Drago P, Falk T, Frenz W: A contactless electromagnetic implantable middle ear device for sensorineural hearing loss. Ear Nose Throat J 1994;73:78–82, 84–88, 90.

10 Hough J, Vernon J, Johnson B, Dormer K, Himelick T: Experiences with implantable hearing devices and a presentation of a new device. Ann Otol Rhinol Laryngol 1986;95:60–65.

11 Fredrickson JM, Coticchia JM, Khosla S: Ongoing investigations into an implantable electromagnetic hearing aid for moderate to severe sensorineural hearing loss. Otolaryngol Clin North Am 1995;28:107–120.

12 Hausler R, Stieger C, Bernhard H, Kompis M: A novel implantable hearing system with direct acoustic cochlear stimulation. Audiol Neurootol 2008;13:247–256.

13 Colletti V, Soli SD, Carner M, Colletti L: Treatment of mixed hearing losses via implantation of a vibratory transducer on the round window. Int J Audiol 2006;45:600–608.

14 Tjellstrom A, Granstrom G: Long-term follow-up with the bone-anchored hearing aid: a review of the first 100 patients between 1977 and 1985. Ear Nose Throat J 1994;73:112–114.

15 Niehaus HH, Helms J, Muller J: Are implantable hearing devices really necessary? Ear Nose Throat J 1995;74:271–274, 276.

16 Todt I, Seidl RO, Gross M, Ernst A: Comparison of different Vibrant Soundbridge audioprocessors with conventional hearing AIDS. Otol Neurotol 2002;23:669–673.

17 Junker R, Gross M, Todt I, Ernst A: Functional gain of already implanted hearing devices in patients with sensorineural hearing loss of varied origin and extent: Berlin experience. Otol Neurotol 2002;23:452–456.

18 Wyatt JR, Niparko JK, Rothman M, deLissovoy G: Cost utility of the multichannel cochlear implants in 258 profoundly deaf individuals. Laryngoscope 1996;106:816–821.

19 Lamden KH, St Leger AS, Raveglia J: Hearing aids: value for money and health gain. J Public Health Med 1995;17:445–449.

20 Snik AF, van Duijnhoven NT, Mylanus EA, Cremers CW: Estimated cost-effectiveness of active middle-ear implantation in hearing-impaired patients with severe external otitis. Arch Otolaryngol Head Neck Surg 2006;132:1210–1215.

21 Ball GR, Huber A, Goode RL: Scanning laser Doppler vibrometry of the middle ear ossicles. Ear Nose Throat J 1997;76:213–218, 220, 222.

22 Tjellstrom A, Luetje CM, Hough JV, Arthur B, Hertzmann P, Katz B, Wallace P: Acute human trial of the floating mass transducer. Ear Nose Throat J 1997;76:204–206, 209–210.

23 Todt I, Seidl RO, Ernst A: Hearing benefit of patients after Vibrant Soundbridge implantation. ORL J Otorhinolaryngol Relat Spec 2005;67:203–206.

24 Luetje CM, Brackman D, Balkany TJ, Maw J, Baker RS, Kelsall D, Backous D, Miyamoto R, Parisier S, Arts A: Phase III clinical trial results with the Vibrant Soundbridge implantable middle ear hearing device: a prospective controlled multicenter study. Otolaryngol Head Neck Surg 2002;126:97–107.

25 Wever EG, Lawrence M: The transmission properties of the middle ear. 1950. Ann Otol Rhinol Laryngol 1992;101:191–204.

26 Wollenberg B, Beltrame M, Schönweiler R, Gehrking E, Nitsch S, Steffen A, Frenzel H: Integration des aktiven Mittelohrimplantates in die plastische Ohrmuschelrekonstruktion. HNO 2007;55:349–356.

27 Hohenhorst W: Classic reconstruction combined with Vibroplasty techniques focused on oval window. International Symposium: Vibroplasty Research, Military Hospital Ulm. September 22nd, 2007.

28 Dumon T: Vibrant Soundbridge middle ear implant in otosclerosis: technique – indication. Adv Otorhinolaryngol 2007;65:320–322.

29 Streitberger C: VSB applied to the oval window and in atresia. Advances in Vibroplasty. Berlin, Unfallkrankenhaus Berlin, 2008.

30 Hüttenbrink KB, Zahnert T, Bornitz M, Beutner D: TORP-vibroplasty: a new alternative for the chronically disabled middle ear. Otol Neurotol 2008;29:965–971.

Prof. A. Ernst
Department of Otolaryngology at ukb
Warener Strasse 7
DE–12683 Berlin (Germany)
Tel. +49 30 5681 4301, Fax +49 30 5681 4303, E-Mail arneborg.ernst@ukb.de

Böheim K (ed): Active Middle Ear Implants.
Adv Otorhinolaryngol. Basel, Karger, 2010, vol 69, pp 27–31

Clinical Results with an Active Middle Ear Implant in the Oval Window

K.B. Hüttenbrink[a] · D. Beutner[a] · T. Zahnert[b]

[a]Department of Otorhinolaryngology, Head and Neck Surgery, University of Cologne, Cologne, and
[b]Technical University of Dresden, Dresden, Germany

Abstract

Background: Some patients with chronic middle ear disease and multiple failed revisions, who also need a hearing aid, may benefit from an active middle ear implant. An advantage of an active middle ear implant is that the ear canal is unoccluded. **Methods:** Following extensive experimental development in temporal bones and investigations of various locations and attachments of a Vibrant Soundbridge transducer, a new titanium clip holder for the vibrant floating mass transducer was developed. This assembly is a total ossicular replacement prosthesis (TORP) that is placed on the stapes footplate. Six patients were implanted with this device. **Results:** Acoustic results demonstrate significantly improved gain, especially in the high frequencies, which is typically unobtainable by conventional hearing aids. **Conclusion:** The simple procedure of placing an active TORP assembly on the stapes footplate, similar to the implantation of a passive TORP prosthesis during tympanoplasty, offers promising treatment for cases of incurable middle ear disease.

Patients with a long history of chronic otitis media often need a hearing aid for communication. This is not only due to unsuccessful restoration of acoustic function of the middle ear despite several tympanoplasty attempts, but also to an often accompanying inner ear hearing loss. Use of a conventional hearing aid ear mold may be uncomfortable because of surgically modified external ear anatomy.

After we developed a hydro-acoustic system that demonstrated the efficiency of direct vibratory stimulation of the inner ear via both round and oval windows [1], we tested the optimal placement of the commercially available Vibrant Soundbridge (VSB) (Vibrant MED-EL, Innsbruck, Austria) in temporal bone experiments. A titanium holder for the floating mass transducer (FMT) was developed in collaboration with the Kurz Company (Dusslingen, Germany). This total ossicular replacement prosthesis (TORP)-FMT assembly was implanted in 6 patients.

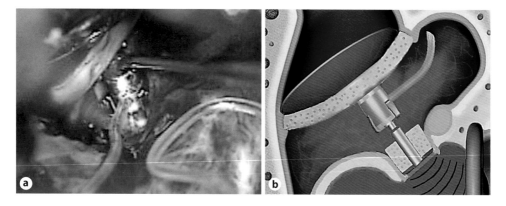

Fig. 1. a Intraoperative view of the assembly with the titanium holder and FMT in its clip, partly covered by the cartilage plate. **b** Schematic illustration of the TORP vibroplasty assembly in the oval window.

Methods

Six patients were implanted, 3 female and 3 male (mean age 67.5 years, range 61–75). The 2 right and 4 left ears had a severely destroyed middle ear with a bare footplate as the sole ossicular remnant, some (4 patients) with a nonfunctional passive TORP lying in the cavity. All patients had bilateral radical cavities with permanent air-bone gaps between 30 and 50 dB and significant (50 dB) inner ear hearing losses. They did not tolerate conventional hearing aids.

After cleaning the oval window niche of granulations and scar tissue, we conducted reconstruction surgery. First, we prepared of a full thickness (1-mm) cartilage shoe with a central hole that was placed in the oval window niche. The rod of our new titanium support was inserted into the central hole and was centered on the footplate. The transducer was inserted into the support by gently pressing it down and fixing it between three clips (fig. 1). The top of the assembly was covered by a cartilage plate – the reconstructed tympanic membrane. In prior radical cavity obliteration cases, the cable was directed out behind the cartilage plates of the partial obliteration to the receiver in its separate bed in the temporalis squama.

Results

Audiometric thresholds, measured 4 weeks after surgery and after removal of ear packing, showed unchanged cochlear function. Figure 2 presents unaided bone conduction thresholds. Unaided air conduction thresholds remained nearly unchanged except in 1 patient, in whom it improved by 20 dB because the inactive assembly works as a passive TORP. Despite increased mass load and friction in the cartilage shoe holder, the average air conduction thresholds in the passive mode were comparable with the situation prior to implantation.

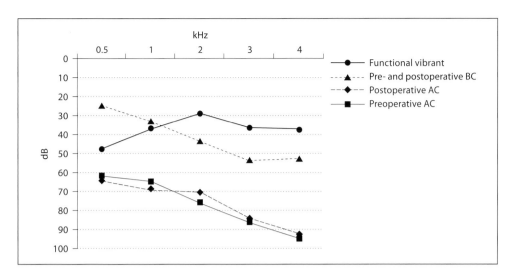

Fig. 2. Pre- and postoperative hearing thresholds of the first 6 patients demonstrating good gain at the high frequencies.

When the VSB was turned on, we observed an improvement of 20 dB in aided soundfield thresholds for frequencies 2 through 4 kHz as compared with bone conduction thresholds (fig. 2).

Good high-frequency gain supported an improvement of monosyllabic word discrimination scores from 0% in the unaided condition to 55% in the VSB-aided condition (average scores, presentation level: 65 dB, Freiburger monosyllabic word discrimination test). According to patients' reports, the improved high-frequency audibility between 2 and 4 kHz was described as a more natural and very pleasant hearing sensation.

Discussion

Contrary to discussions on indications for implantable hearing aids in sensorineural hearing loss [2], their benefit in patients with permanently defect middle ear and unsatisfactory audiologic results with passive prostheses is demonstrated in an increasing number of successful implantations throughout the world [3–5]. The ear canal remains open, and the conductive component of the hearing loss is bypassed. Improvement in aided hearing thresholds, especially at high frequencies, is an important advantage. The alternative treatment, a bone-anchored hearing aid, is limited in cases of severe cochlear dysfunction because of limited amplification. For our patients, the surgical intervention was accepted because they had tolerated several revision tympanoplasties well in the past and had asked for additional revision tympanoplasty to improve their hearing.

We analyzed the optimal position for the VSB FMT in the inner ear in our temporal bone experiments prior to clinical use [6]. Direct contact to the stapes footplate gives better performance, especially for high frequencies between 2 and 4 kHz because of the large vibrating area of the complete footplate. Furthermore, the surgical procedure for the placement on the footplate might be seen as less demanding compared to the round window niche placement. Insertion into the round window niche often requires drilling the bony overhang with the risk of cochlear trauma [7]. This is due to restrictions in the approach, anatomical variations, and the relatively large diameter of the FMT (1.6 mm) as compared to the opening of the round window niche (1.3–1.6 mm) [8, 9]. Furthermore, permanently stable contact with the inner ear fluid, while also avoiding any hard contact to the surrounding bone, is mandatory for efficient coupling. A loose contact between the FMT and the round window membrane/cochlear fluid results in reduced amplification. Mechanical restriction might explain the variable acoustic results reported in the literature on the round window placement. In some cases, the aided thresholds did not surpass the bone conduction thresholds [10].

Inconsistent contact of the FMT is avoided when the FMT is placed in direct contact with the footplate. Due to limited space in the oval window niche, a titanium holder was required. Secure attachment to the stapes footplate, preventing any lateral displacement, is assured when our cartilage shoe technique for the passive TORP procedure is used [11]. The FMT is attached to the support by modifying the clip design of our Clip-partial ossicular replacement prosthesis (PORP) [12]. In cases of an intact stapes, two clips (one for the FMT and the other for the stapes head) form the PORP design. Therefore, by using the developments for passive prostheses and by closing the tympanic cavity with a thick cartilage plate, stable assembly anchorage to the footplate is established.

Our first audiologic results support data gathered in our temporal bone experiments and demonstrate good acoustic benefit of directly coupling the FMT to the stapes footplate. Amplification of 40–60 dB in the high frequencies would not be possible with a conventional air conduction hearing aid. The surgical procedure, about as simple as the placement of a conventional TORP on the footplate, is another advantage over drilling the round window niche and the risk of inconsistent transducer placement in contact with the membrane.

Because the TORP also provides hearing benefit when used passively, patients with a moderate hearing loss might use active stimulation only in noisy or demanding listening situations (e.g. parties). Therefore, this TORP- (or future PORP-) supported VSB assembly can be offered to a large group of patients with permanently damaged middle ear function and additional sensorineural hearing loss, who are not candidates for conventional hearing aids or bone-anchored hearing aids. A good hearing prognosis can be offered to these patients with a simple and modified 'active tympanoplasty procedure'.

References

1 Hüttenbrink KB: Biomechanical aspects in implantable microphones and hearing aids and development of a concept with a hydroacoustical transmission. Acta Otolarnygol 2001;121:185–189.

2 Hüttenbrink KB: Current status and critical reflexions on implantable hearing aids. Am J Otol 1999; 20:409–415.

3 Coletti V, Soli SD, Carner M, Colletti L: Treatment of mixed hearing losses via implantation of a vibratory transducer on the round window. Int J Audiol 2006;45:600–608.

4 Kiefer J: Round Window Stimulation with an Implantable Hearing Aid Soundbridge® combined with autogenous reconstruction of the auricle: a new approach. ORL 2006;68:375–385.

5 Wollenberg B: Integration of the active middle ear implant in total auricular reconstruction (in German). HNO 2007;55:349–356.

6 Hüttenbrink KB, Zahnert Th, Bornitz M, Beutner D: TORP-vibroplasty: a new alternative for the chronically disabled middle ear. Otol Neurotol 2008;29:965–971.

7 Pau HW, Just T, Bornitz M, Lasurashvilli M, Zahnert Th: Noise exposure of the inner ear during drilling a cochleostomy for cochlear implantation. Laryngoscope 2007;117:535–540.

8 Nomura Y: Otological significances of the round window. Adv Otorhinolaryngol 1984;33:11–99.

9 Roland MD: Cochlear implant electrode insertion: the round window revisited. Laryngoscope 2007; 117:1397–1402.

10 Soli S: Comparison of output levels and gains for bone conduction and round window stimulation of the cochlea in patients with conductive hearing loss. Proc 5th Int Symp on Human Sensibility Recovery Systems, Kyungpook National University Daegu, Korea, 2007.

11 Hüttenbrink KB, Zahnert T, Beutner D, Hofmann G: The cartilage guide: a solution for anchoring a columella prosthesis on footplate (in German). Laryngorhinootologie 2004;83:450–456.

12 Hüttenbrink KB, Zahnert Th, Wüstenberg E, Hofmann G: Titanium clip prosthesis. Otol Neurotol 2004;25:436–442.

Prof. Dr. K. B. Hüttenbrink
HNO-Uniklinik Köln
Kerpener Strasse 60
DE–50937 Köln (Germany)
Tel. +49 221 478 4750, Fax +49 221 478 4793
E-Mail huettenbrink.k-b@uni-koeln.de

Böheim K (ed): Active Middle Ear Implants.
Adv Otorhinolaryngol. Basel, Karger, 2010, vol 69, pp 32–37

Experiments on the Coupling of an Active Middle Ear Implant to the Stapes Footplate

T. Zahnert[a] · M. Bornitz[a] · K.B. Hüttenbrink[b]

[a]Department of Otorhinolaryngology, University Clinic of Dresden, Dresden, and
[b]University Clinic of Cologne, Cologne, Germany

Abstract

Background: Although the function of active middle ear implants in cases of intact ossicular chains and ventilated middle ears is well known, information about sound transfer function to the inner ear in cases of chronic middle ear effusion and defective middle ear structures is needed. A temporal bone model was developed to measure (1) the coupling of the active middle ear implant Vibrant Soundbridge in cases of nonventilated radical cavities, and (2) the effect of effusion and cartilage shielding. **Methods:** Three fresh human temporal bone specimens were studied. After preparation of a radical cavity, the floating mass transducer was coupled to the stapes footplate. The transducer was stimulated with 50 mV multisinus signals and inner ear fluid vibration was measured using a microphone in the round window niche. Several coupling conditions were simulated with mass and stiffness variations and cartilage shielding. **Results:** Coupling modality and prestress have the most influence on the sound transfer function to the inner ear. Cartilage shielding may ensure better coupling of the FMT to the footplate. The effect of middle ear effusion is negligible. **Conclusion:** The Vibrant Soundbridge provides good sound transfer to the inner ear not only in cases of coupling onto an intact ossicular chain in a ventilated middle ear but also in cases of coupling to the stapes footplate in non-ventilated radical cavities.

Passive middle ear implants provide good hearing results in middle ears that are normally ventilated with healthy tympanic membranes when there is no or only a moderate air-bone gap. Active middle ear implants (AMEIs) are traditionally indicated for persons with moderate-to-severe sensorineural hearing loss, an intact ossicular chain, and normal middle ear ventilation. The electromagnetic transducer of the Vibrant Soundbridge (VSB) has been successfully implanted and good hearing results in a large number of patients have been demonstrated, especially in the high-frequency

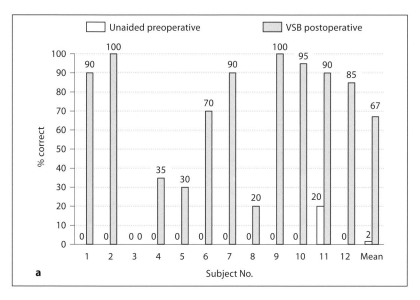

a

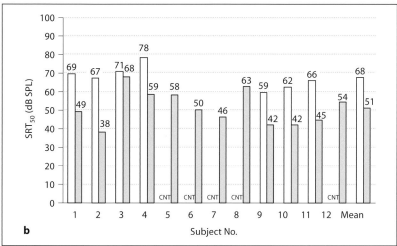

b

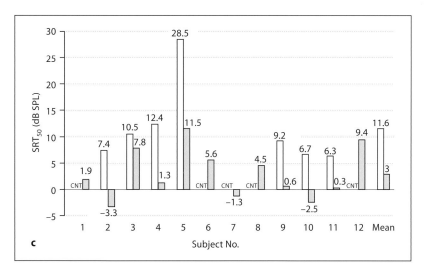

c

postoperative data and shows that 11 of 12 subjects were unable to score above 0% preoperatively whereas almost all were able to score better than 0% postoperatively aided with the VSB, with the majority of subjects scoring better than 70% correct. Sentence recognition in quiet showed an improvement in OLSA thresholds for 50% correct recognition from 68 dB SPL (SD = 6) preoperatively to 51 dB SPL (SD = 9) postoperatively. Figure 2b presents individual results and shows that SRT_{50} ranged from about 38 to 68 dB SPL postoperatively for all subjects, although 5 subjects were unable to complete the test preoperatively. Sentence recognition in noise (mean OLSA SNRs for 50% correct recognition presented in background noise) improved from +12 dB SPL SNR (SD = 8) preoperatively to 3 dB SPL SNR (SD = 5) postoperatively (fig. 2c).

Subjective Benefits
Significant changes in self-reported hearing performance from the unaided to the VSB-aided condition were observed as reductions in the percentage of problems on ease of communication (mean pre- to postoperative 66 to 28%, p = 0.001), Reverberation (mean pre- to postoperative 72 to 43%, p = 0.005), and background noise (mean pre- to postoperative 73 to 40%, p = 0.002) subscales of the APHAB. The aversiveness subscale showed no significant change (mean pre- to postoperative 30 to 35%, p > 0.05). Significant improvement in overall device satisfaction was demonstrated in a mean improvement from 43% (SD = 28.7) preoperatively to 74% (SD = 18.5) postoperatively (p = 0.005) on the HDSS. Changes in QoL attributed to VSB use were observed in the areas of overall benefit and general benefit, which showed average positive changes of 17 and 24, respectively. The areas of social benefit and physical benefit showed much less change, changing an average of –6 and 11, respectively.

Changes in Residual Hearing
Changes in unaided hearing were evaluated by comparing preoperative unaided BC hearing thresholds with postoperative BC thresholds for audiometric test frequencies 500 through 4,000 Hz. There were no significant changes at any frequency (p > 0.05). Air conduction thresholds were also unchanged (p > 0.05). Figure 1a presents mean pre- and postoperative air and BC thresholds.

Medical and Surgical Complications
One subject (No. 3) required surgery to improve coupling between the FMT and the RW membrane. The subject initially experienced device benefit but performance declined rapidly following initial device fitting. Surgery for repositioning took place after the subject concluded study participation and data included here were collected before the second surgery (e.g. the subject's data, reflecting poorer performance, are included). Audiologic performance and hearing benefit were reportedly good following the repositioning surgery. No other major medical or surgical complications were reported.

Böheim K (ed): Active Middle Ear Implants.
Adv Otorhinolaryngol. Basel, Karger, 2010, vol 69, pp 51–58

Clinical Experience with the Active Middle Ear Implant Vibrant Soundbridge in Sensorineural Hearing Loss

S.M. Pok · M. Schlögel · K. Böheim

Department of Otorhinolaryngology, Head and Neck Surgery, Landesklinikum St. Pölten, St. Pölten, Österreich

Abstract

Background/Aims: To evaluate gain at threshold level and speech recognition performance of 54 subjects with mild-to-severe symmetrical sensorineural hearing loss (SNHL) that received the active middle ear implant system Vibrant Soundbridge (VSB). *Methods:* Pre- and postoperative assessments of hearing thresholds and monosyllabic word discrimination were performed in a homogeneous group of 54 adults who received a VSB system (VORP 502/AP 404) in an active middle ear implant (AMEI) program in a tertiary referral hospital. All subjects included in this study had mild-to-severe, predominately sloping SNHL. Gain at threshold level and speech recognition results were assessed for unaided and aided conditions using the patient's walk-in hearing aid (HA) and the VSB in a retrospective study design. *Results:* A comparison of pre- and postoperative unaided air conduction thresholds revealed a mean decrease in pure tone averages of 3.9 dB (0.25–8 kHz). Gain at threshold level (unaided thresholds minus AMEI-aided thresholds) was, on average, 20.9 dB at 0.5 kHz, 20.5 dB at 1 kHz, 23.8 dB at 2 kHz, 30.2 dB at 3 kHz, 36.1 dB at 4 kHz, 37.6 dB at 6 kHz and 37.9 dB at 8 kHz. Monosyllabic word discrimination at 65 dB SPL improved from a mean of 30% in the unaided condition to 44% for the HA-aided condition (p < 0.05), with a further increase to 57% for the VSB-aided condition (p < 0.05, compared to the HA). *Conclusion:* The AMEI system VSB can be considered as an effective rehabilitation alternative in subjects with mild-to-severe SNHL and unsatisfying benefit from conventional hearing aids.

Active middle ear implants (AMEI) have been available to treat sensorineural hearing loss (SNHL) for more than a decade. A number of studies demonstrated the safety and effectiveness of several types of AMEIs in the last years [1–7]. Substantial experience has been gained with the Vibrant Soundbridge (VSB; MED-EL, Innsbruck, Austria) which has been proven to be a safe, appropriate and cost-effective rehabilitation alternative for patients with SNHL who are unable to achieve adequate benefit or are medically unable to tolerate conventional hearing aids (HAs) [2, 7, 8]. Previous studies reported improvements in overall sound quality, clarity of sound and tone quality: they also indicated high satisfaction scores with the VSB as a treatment for SNHL [6, 9]. Several comparative studies of the VSB in high-frequency SNHL found better speech recognition scores with the AMEI as compared with several types of conventional HAs [10–13].

In recent years, alternative techniques for coupling for the transducer to the middle ear have been developed. For example, the round-window technique or a floating mass transducer-total ossicular replacement prosthesis (FMT-TORP), which allows the VSB indication to be extended to conductive and mixed hearing losses [14–17]. However, the VSB was originally designed for use in SNHL using an incus coupling of the FMT to the intact ossicular chain. The incus application bypasses both the ear canal and the tympanic membrane and reduces acoustic feedback. In addition, the occlusion effect and ear canal distortions that occur at high acoustic amplification levels are minimized. In the frequency range above 4 kHz, the FMT's frequency response delivers more maximum amplification as compared with the maximum output that can be realized with conventional HAs.

In the HA literature, it is controversially discussed whether or not high-frequency audibility is beneficial to speech recognition [18, 19]. Many studies found no significant improvement or significant benefit only in background noise, whereas other authors found improvements in quiet and noise, as well as in other auditory abilities, such as spatial hearing, HA acceptance, and sound quality. In the AMEI literature, authors have suggested that stable high-frequency amplification via direct drive of the ossicular chain might contribute to improved speech recognition, especially in noise [10, 11, 20]. Unfortunately, AMEI studies only sporadically report on VSB-aided pure tone hearing thresholds for the high-frequency range above 4 kHz; published data in the extended frequency range from 6 to 8 kHz are very rare. Only three studies reported VSB-aided thresholds in the frequency range of 6–8 kHz in a few subjects [10, 12, 20].

The aim of this study is to evaluate gain at the threshold level and speech recognition performance in 54 subjects with mild-to-severe symmetrical SNHL. All subjects received a VSB system at an implant program in an ear-nose-throat clinic in a tertiary referral hospital. We assessed pre- and postoperative hearing thresholds (0.25–8 kHz) in the unaided and the VSB-aided condition. In addition, speech recognition performance in unaided, HA and VSB conditions was evaluated.

Methods

Study Design
A within-subjects, retrospective study design was used to assess audiologic status and performance before and after implantation of the VSB.

Pok · Schlögel · Böheim

In general, our findings on unaided and aided hearing thresholds show that the VSB system provides substantial and stable amplification up to the high frequencies and allows an adequate treatment in SNHL within the entire recommended indication field.

Regarding speech recognition results, an audiologic benefit for both device types, the HA and the AMEI, as compared with the unaided condition, was found. When comparing aided conditions, monosyllabic word recognition with the AMEI was significantly better than with the subjects' walk-in HA. Subjects with hearing losses near and at the lower limit of the recommended indication field also received benefit from the VSB system. Other authors found similar improvements when comparing the VSB with different types of HAs. Uziel et al. [10] attributed the benefit to superior sound transmission quality via direct-drive stimulation. In that comparative study, the authors assessed the hearing benefit for patients with high-frequency hearing loss obtained from an AMEI and a conventional hearing aid using the same hearing aid processing circuitry. According to their measurements, significant advantages for speech discrimination in quiet and in noise in favor of the AMEI were found, despite similar amounts of gain for the study HA and the VSB.

The data demonstrate the potential benefit of vibromechanical stimulation in cases of SNHL with unsatisfactory benefit from conventional HA. This is also reflected in the high rate of device acceptance: in our 54 subjects, 36 used a HA prior to surgery and 18 subjects (or 33%) were HA owners but permanent nonusers despite multiple adequate attempts of conventional HA rehabilitation. In contrast, all of them adopted their AMEI immediately after the first fitting and use their device on a daily basis.

Conclusion

In cases of SNHL with unsatisfying benefit from conventional HAs, the VSB system offers an attractive and effective hearing solution.

References

1 Zenner HP, Leysieffer H: Total implantation of the Implex TICA hearing amplifier implant for high frequency sensorineural hearing loss: the Tübingen University experience. Otolaryngol Clin North Am 2001;34:417–446.

2 Mosnier I, Sterkers O, Bouccara D, et al: Benefit of the Vibrant Soundbridge device in patients implanted for 5 to 8 years. Ear Hear 2008;29:281–284.

3 Lenarz T, Weber BP, Issing PR, et al: The Vibrant Soundbridge: a new kind of hearing aid for sensorineural hearing loss. 2. Audiological results. Laryngorhinootologie 2001;80:370–380.

4 Kasic JF, Fredrickson JM: The Otologics MET ossicular stimulator. Otolaryngol Clin North Am 2001;34:501–513.

5 Snik AF, Mylanus EA, Cremers CW, et al: Multicenter audiometric results with the Vibrant Soundbridge, a semi-implantable hearing device for sensorineural hearing impairment. Otolaryngol Clin North Am 2001;34:373–388.

6 Sterkers O, Boucarra D, Labassi S, et al: A middle ear implant, the Symphonix Vibrant Soundbridge: retrospective study of the first 125 patients implanted in France. Otol Neurotol 2003;24:427–436.

7 Schmuziger N, Schimmann F, àWengen D, Patscheke J, Probst R: Long-term assessment after implantation of the Vibrant Soundbridge device. Otol Neurotol 2006;27:183–188.

8 Snik AF, van Duijnhoven NT, Mylanus EA, Cremers CW: Estimated cost-effectiveness of active middle-ear implantation in hearing-impaired patients with severe external otitis. Arch Otolaryngol Head Neck Surg 2006;132:1210–1215.

9 Luetje CM, Brackman D, Balkany TJ, et al: Phase III clinical trial results with the Vibrant Soundbridge implantable middle ear hearing device: a prospective controlled multicenter study. Otolaryngol Head Neck Surg 2002;126:97–107.

10 Uziel A, Mondain M, Hagen P, Dejean F, Doucet G: Rehabilitation for high-frequency sensorineural hearing impairment in adults with the Symphonix Vibrant Soundbridge: a comparative study. Otol Neurotol 2003;24:775–783.

11 Truy E, Philibert B, Vesson JF, Labassi S, Collet L: Vibrant Soundbridge versus conventional hearing aid in sensorineural high-frequency hearing loss: a prospective study. Otol Neurotol 2008;29:684–687.

12 Todt I, Seidl RO, Gross M, Ernst A: Comparison of different Vibrant Soundbridge audioprocessors with conventional hearing aids. Otol Neurotol 2002;23:669–673.

13 Boeheim K, Pok SM, Schloegel M, Filzmoser P: Active middle ear implant compared with open-fit hearing aid in sloping high-frequency sensorineural hearing loss. Otol Neurotol 2010;31:424–429.

14 Colletti V, Soli SD, Carner M, Colletti L: Treatment of mixed hearing losses via implantation of a vibratory transducer on the round window. Int J Audiol 2006;45:600–608.

15 Huber AM, Ball GR, Veraguth D, Dillier N, Bodmer D, Sequeira D: A new implantable middle ear hearing device for mixed hearing loss: a feasibility study in human temporal bones. Otol Neurotol 2006;27:1104–1109.

16 Beltrame A, Martini A, Prosser S, Giarbini N, Streitberger C: Coupling the Vibrant Soundbridge to cochlea round window: auditory results in patients with mixed hearing loss. Otol Neurotol 2009;30:194–201.

17 Frenzel H, Hanke F, Beltrame M, Steffen A, Schönweiler R, Wollenberg B: Application of the Vibrant Soundbridge to unilateral osseous atresia cases. Laryngoscope 2009;119:67–74.

18 Amos NE, Humes LE: Contribution of high frequencies to speech recognition in quiet and noise in listeners with varying degrees of high-frequency sensorineural hearing loss. J Speech Lang Hear Res 2007;50:819–834.

19 Baer T, Moore BC, Kluk K: Effects of low pass filtering on the intelligibility of speech in noise for people with and without dead regions at high frequencies. J Acoust Soc Am 2002;112:1133–1144.

20 Böheim K, Nahler A, Schlögel M: Rehabilitation of high frequency hearing loss: use of an active middle ear implant. HNO 2007;55:690–695.

21 Sandlin R: Textbook of Hearing Aid Amplification, Technical and Clinical Considerations, ed 2. San Diego, Singular Publishing Group, 2000, pp 82–86.

22 Hahlbrock K-H: Sprachaudiometrie, ed 2. Stuttgart, Thieme, 1970.

23 Hollander M, Wolfe DA: Nonparametric Statistical Inference. New York, Wiley, 1973.

24 Needham AJ, Jiang D, Bibas A, Jeronimidis G, O'Connor P, Fitzgerald A: The effects of mass loading the ossicles with a floating mass transducer on middle ear transfer function. Otol Neurotol 2005;26:218–224.

25 Schmuziger N, Probst R, Smurzynski J: Test-retest reliability of pure-tone thresholds from 0.5 to 16 kHz using Sennheiser HDA 200 and Etymotic Research ER-2 earphones. Ear Hear 2004;25:127–132.

26 Snik AF, Mylanus EA, Cremers CW, Dillier N, Fisch U, Gnadeberg D, Lenarz T, Mazolli M, Babighian G, Uziel AS, Cooper HR, O'Connor AF, Fraysse B, Charachon R, Shehata-Dieler WE: Multicenter audiometric results with the Vibrant Soundbridge, a semi-implantable hearing device for sensorineural hearing impairment. Otolaryngol Clin North Am 2001;34:373–388.

27 Vibrant Soundbridge, The Middle Ear Implant System: Document No. 28066, Data Sheet p14, printed by Vibrant Med-El Hearing Technology GmbH, Innsbruck, Austria, 2009.

28 Glasberg B, Moore B: Auditory filter shapes in subjects with unilateral and bilateral cochlear impairments. J Acoust Soc Am 1986;79:1020–1033.

Prof. Klaus Boeheim
Department of Otorhinolaryngology, Head and Neck Surgery
Landesklinikum St. Pölten
Propst Fuehrerstrasse 4
AT–3100 St. Pölten (Austria)
Tel. +43 2742 300 12901, Fax +43 2742 300 12919
E-Mail Klaus.Boeheim@stpoelten.lknoe.at

Böheim K (ed): Active Middle Ear Implants.
Adv Otorhinolaryngol. Basel, Karger, 2010, vol 69, pp 59–71

The Esteem System:
A Totally Implantable Hearing Device

J. Maurer · E. Savvas

Department for Otorhinolaryngolgy, Head and Neck Surgery, and Center for Hearing and Communication, Katholisches Klinikum Koblenz, Koblenz, Germany

Abstract

The Esteem totally implantable active middle ear implant is a new technology to augment hearing in patients suffering from moderate-to-severe and severe sensorineural hearing loss. In contrast to conventional (acoustic) hearing aids, the system uses two piezoelectric transducers (PZTs). PZTs are used as the sensor and driver to replace the function of the middle ear. Sound is received via a PZT sensor that picks up eardrum vibrations, following the piezoelectric principle, and transforms them into an electric signal. This signal is filtered, modified, amplified and transferred to a PZT driver, which mechanically drives the stapes and thereby the inner ear. The sound processor also contains a power source, which is an implantable lithium iodide battery. All components of the hearing restoration system are totally implantable to offer good sound fidelity and reduce hearing aid stigma caused by the visibility of conventional and semi-implantable hearing systems. Our experience shows that this system can provide considerable benefit to patients with sensorineural hearing loss.

System Concept and Background

There is accumulating evidence supporting the principle of directly driving the ossicular chain as a means of providing amplification and good sound transmission to hearing impaired patients.

The Esteem system concept is based on two piezoelectric transducers (PZTs): one placed on the incus and the other placed on the stapes. The first transducer (the sensor, fig. 1a, b) detects tympanic membrane motion in response to sound via the malleus on the incus. The sound signal is then processed by the processor (fig. 1a, b) to

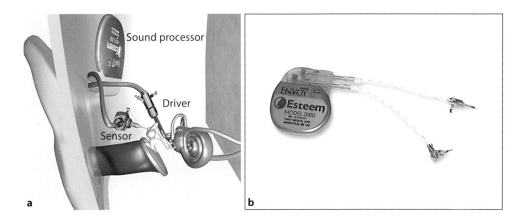

Fig. 1. a The Esteem implanted system components. **b** The Esteem implantable components.

meet the patient's hearing loss and is used to drive a second PZT (the driver, fig. 1a, b) placed on the stapes. This vibrates the stapes and mechanical vibration is detected as sound in the cochlea. To prevent feedback, the incus is separated from the stapes at the level of the incudostapedial joint and 1–2 mm of the long process is resected during device placement. Success is dependent on two key principles: the reversible electromechanical properties of piezoelectric ceramics and the proven benefits of directly driving the ossicular chain. The Esteem System (Envoy Medical Corporation, St. Paul, Minn., USA) carries the CE marking in Europe since 2006.

PZT Sensor and Driver

Piezoelectric materials have the property of reversible electromechanical transduction. When a force is applied to the material, voltage is generated and, conversely, when voltage is applied, motion is created. This property is most efficient when the ceramic is formed in the shape of a cantilever (diving board) with one end fixed and the other end mobile. This results in the greatest displacement for an applied voltage. Each PZT consists of two internal plates of a PZT crystal aggregate of $PbZr_xTi_xO_3$, and the configuration is known as a bimorph. The plates can be connected in series or in parallel. When the sensor transducer plates are connected in series, a greater voltage is generated; when the driver transducer plates are connected in parallel, a greater displacement for an applied voltage is generated.

The sensor PZT is similar to a microphone in a conventional hearing aid. A conventional microphone consists of a diaphragm and a ceramic element. The diaphragm serves to collect sound over a large area. The motion of the diaphragm is detected by the ceramic element and converted to a voltage. In the Esteem, the microphone is replaced by the PZT sensor and is placed on the incus. The tympanic membrane acts as

Maurer · Savvas

the diaphragm, collecting sound over a far greater area than the sensor alone. In addition, the tympanic membrane is situated at the most medial end of the ear canal, which is advantageous. The external auditory canal acts as a filter, giving stronger emphasis to high-frequency than to low-frequency sounds [1]. The amplification provided by the ear canal is as much as 10 × (20 dB) and is greatest at frequencies 1 through 4 kHz. Low-frequency sounds are amplified minimally or not at all.

The relative effect of sound filtration is determined both by the frequency and the incident direction of the sound. Placing any microphone or the Envoy PZT sensor at the tympanic membrane provides a natural filtration benefit. The PZT sensor is fastened to the wall of the mastoid with cement to fix one end, while the motion of the incus vibrates the other end (the sensor tip). Sensor output is relatively constant across frequencies, and around 1,000 Hz it begins to roll off. A similar roll-off is seen in stapes displacement. Because the stapes and malleus/incus displacements roll off at a similar rate, the driver output at any one frequency is a direct function of the sensor input at the same frequency. The processes of amplification, filtration, and compression are adjusted to compensate for the patient's particular hearing loss.

The PZT driver is fastened to the wall of the mastoid with cement to fix one end, while the motion of the PZT driver vibrates the stapes via attachment to the stapes head with a microscopic drop of glass ionomer cement with zero bias. When a voltage is applied to the driver transducer, the tip of the cantilever displaces the stapes.

There is a theoretical advantage of directly driving the ossicular chain. This concept has been developed over many years with encouraging results. Wilska, in 1935, placed pieces of soft iron on the tympanic membrane, and, under the influence of an electromagnetic field, subjects were able to perceive tones. In the 1970s and 1980s, magnets were placed on the stapes and speech conduction tested.

Yanagihara et al. [2] developed a partially implantable device, which was successfully used in over 60 subjects but suffered from insufficient acoustic output. It consisted of an external microphone and an internal piezoelectric driver placed on the stapes. Implanted patients showed some encouraging trends, especially in speech discrimination results. Kodera et al. [3], in a study of 6 implanted patients, demonstrated improved performance for both speech and music when compared with a conventional hearing aid. Speech discrimination scores were 10% better than with conventional hearing aids in the same patients. Testing in an environment with competing background noise, this difference was statistically significant at the 0.05 level. Similar results were reported by Suzuki et al. [4]. The active middle ear implant was superior to a conventional hearing aid in the perception of speech, music, and environmental sounds. Patients preferred the fidelity of sound, claiming it was more natural sounding than their hearing aids.

Active middle ear implant results have been very encouraging; however, the number of patients with speech discrimination data was small and all patients had had only mild or moderate hearing losses. Patients with more severe hearing losses, likely candidates for the Esteem, tend to have greater difficulties with impaired speech discrimination and recruitment. The Esteem system increases the efficiency of sound reaching the inner ear, which may aid in improved speech discrimination. However, it does not improve cochlear or eighth nerve function; therefore, the impressive gains of the Japanese device may be less evident in a more compromised population.

In a 1973 study of directly driving the ossicular chain, Goode and Glattke [5] noted that patients preferred speech presented through a magnet attached to the ossicular chain to speech presented through a conventional audiometer. No improvement in speech discrimination scores was reported. This may be because only quiet and not noisy background conditions were tested. The Japanese group noted the greatest improvement in a noisy environment.

Mahoney and Vernon [6] recorded cochlear microphonics, which can be played through loudspeakers and recognized as sound. Using a hearing impaired guinea pig, they initially presented speech to the animal's ear through a conventional hearing aid and then by directly driving the ossicular chain with a piezoelectric crystal. The cochlear microphonic was recorded and played back to normal hearing listeners who were asked to identify the words. Discrimination scores were 16% better in normal hearing adults when the ossicular chain was directly driven, which might suggest that the quality of information being received by the inner ear is better when the chain is directly driven.

The reason for the possible sound quality improvement with direct-drive stimulation could relate to the impedance of air. A conventional hearing aid detects sound, which is processed, amplified and then played via a loudspeaker. This loudspeaker moves a cushion of air, sitting between the speaker and the ear drum. This is an inefficient process. Transient sounds are not conducted well, and the presence of the hearing aid in the external canal occludes the ear and prevents natural filtering. In newer aids with an open ear canal, some acoustic energy is lost because the open ear canal is open. Directly driving the ossicular chain potentially allows more efficient sound transmission to the ossicles. Transient sounds are more efficiently conducted, and because the ear canal is unoccluded, less acoustic gain is required than with a conventional aid.

Studies of the Vibrant Soundbridge demonstrated the benefits of directly driving the ossicular chain. Patients preferred the sound quality and found hearing in noisy environments easier than with conventional hearing aids [7]. The data were supported by the observations of Maassen et al. [8] with direct vibration of the ossicular chain.

One can conclude that by directly driving the ossicular chain:
(1) mechanically induced sounds have the same characteristics as their acoustic counterparts,
(2) in patients with mild-to-moderate hearing losses, there is a possible improvement in speech discrimination compared with a conventional hearing aid, and
(3) speech discrimination improvements are most evident for speech in noise, music, and environmental sounds.

Sound Processor

To optimize the PZT sensor input and the PZT driver output, a series of electronic circuits is required. These are contained within a titanium enclosure, the sound processor (fig. 1a, b). The sound processor also contains a battery to power the circuits, which are mostly contained within an application-specific integrated circuit and perform audio signal processing and digital telemetric functions.

Sound vibrates the tympanic membrane, which moves the PZT sensor. A small generated voltage is conducted along the lead wires into the header, which is the connector block attached to the sound processor into which the leads connect (similar to a pacemaker). The signal then passes into the application-specific integrated circuit, where it is separated into two channels and filtered. Compression is applied to optimize the available dynamic range. The signal is amplified to achieve acoustic parity and compensate for the patient's particular hearing impairment. The output signal passes out of the header to the PZT driver lead wire. This signal oscillates the driver, moving the stapes in response to sound.

The use of piezoelectric materials and a low-power circuit design allow an expected battery life of 6–9 years, depending on individual patient programming and daily usage. A bi-directional telemetric circuit controls the amplifier circuitry, tones generated, and device programming. Within the titanium can is a loop antenna, which receives and transmits binary control codes. Commands from programmer are downloaded to the device, and changes within the memory are made. Synthesized tones from an internal tone generator are used to measure hearing thresholds, volume setting, program selection, and compression ratio and knee point settings in the channels. Tonal confirmation of any parameter change is provided. The state of the device memory, device serial number and other parameters can also be uploaded to the programmer. Multiple redundant protection mechanisms exist within the telemetric circuitry so that aberrant codes do not alter device performance. Each implanted device has a unique electronic access code, providing a further measure of security.

The lead wires within the body may act as an antenna, detecting stray radiofrequency signals generated from cellular telephones, microwaves, and many other electronic devices. These signals can interfere with the signals entering the system, potentially leading to sound degradation or to other unwanted noise. To overcome this effect, the titanium case is laser welded hermetically shut, and all leads entering or exiting the case pass through broadband electromagnetic interference (EMI) discoidal filters. These discoidal filters are continuous with the case and are effective in removing the 10 MHz to 10 GHz signals presented by most appliances and cellular telephones.

Indications

Patients should have a sensorineural hearing impairment and be 18 years or older at the time of implantation. In addition, they should have had experience with hearing

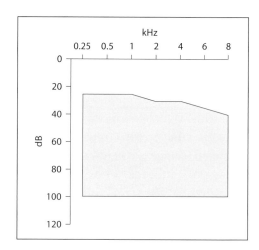

Fig. 2. Audiological inclusion criteria.

aids. Hearing thresholds should be stable and between 35 and 85 dB HL for audiometric test frequencies of 500–4,000 Hz with a word recognition score of 40% or greater (unaided, Freiburg monosyllabic word test). The audiometric indication field is shown in figure 2. Retrocochlear hearing loss should be ruled out. A CT scan should show a mastoid large enough to accommodate the sensor and driver.

Surgical Procedure

The surgical procedure generally follows the techniques used for cochlear implantation, the main difference being that the inner ear remains untouched. The PZT sensor and the PZT driver are attached to the ossicular chain. After incising the skin, subcutaneous and muscle flaps are formed and a mastoidectomy is carried out. A bone bed is then drilled out to accommodate the sound processor, and a tunnel is created for the cable link. The ossicular chain, especially the long process of the incus and the stapes, can be fully exposed via posterior tympanotomy. A CO_2 laser is used to remove 2 mm of the long process of the incus, including the lenticular process.

The PZT sensor is fixed to the superior edge of the mastoidectomy with the tip positioned onto the incus body. The PZT driver is attached to the inferior edge of the mastoidectomy and its tip positioned onto the exposed stapes head. The sound processor is fixed into the bone bed. The wound is closed after intraoperative testing of the whole system using laser Doppler vibrometry and, optionally, acoustic brainstem audiometry.

Preparation of the Patient

Surgery is performed with the patient lying in a horizontal position with the head turned to the side contralateral to implantation. After shaving the incision area, local anesthetics with adrenaline are applied, facial nerve monitoring is installed, and the skin is disinfected. The patient's head is covered with sterile drapes.

The incision must always be a minimum distance of 1 cm from the implant. It is made at the beginning of the mastoid tip at a distance of 1 cm of the retroauricular fold, which turns craniodorsally approximately 2 cm above the ear. The subcutaneous-muscle-periost flap is prepared dorsally and the pericranium is elevated further to accommodate the processor. Hemostasis must be carefully performed to minimize the use of bipolar cautery after positioning the implant.

The mastoid plane, the temporal line, and the mastoid tip are exposed and the external auditory canal identified. The mastoid is drilled out to accommodate the PZT sensor and PZT driver. The bone covering the middle and posterior cranial fossae, the sigmoid sinus up to the mastoid tip, the labyrinth with its horizontal and posterior semicircular duct, the antrum with the incus, and the osseous canal of the facial nerve in the mastoid is thinned out. The posterior wall of the external auditory canal is then thinned until all cells are removed. The surrounding bone at the incus site must be completely removed in order to have wide access to the area around the antrum. The wall of the external auditory canal may be thinned in this process. The osseous cells in the direction of the middle cranial fossa are also drilled out.

Approximately 1 cm behind and above the mastoidectomy, a bone bed is created for the sound processor. A plane osseous area on the occipital bone and temporal bone is selected to achieve a flat bone bed. The bone bed is drilled out. Irregularities must be removed in order to prevent the implant from rocking. Usually, it is not necessary to expose the dura. The sound processor is later fixed in the bone bed with crossed resorbable sutures or by tightly suturing the pericranium and the muscle-skin flap over the processor and thereby fixing the implant.

A posterior tympanotomy is performed with diamond drills of various sizes between 4 and 1.5 mm under an operating microscope. The tip of the short process of the incus, as well as the osseous course of the facial nerve, can provide orientation. Near the tip of the incus, the bone must be removed carefully while adhering to the course of the facial nerve until the first cells are reached in the direction of the middle ear. The bone of the posterior wall of the external auditory canal must be thinned carefully to expose the course of the chorda tympani. The angle of the chorda tympani and the facial nerve is then enlarged and the bone removed until the posterior tympanotomy is extended as far caudally and cranially as possible. The bone in the direction of the tympanic sinus should also be removed. If possible, the entire stapes should be visible from the footplate to the head. It is important to make sure that the drill does not touch the tip of the incus. This preparation is crucial for positioning and fixation of the driver.

The ossicular chain must be interrupted to avoid feedback between the PZT sensor and the PZT driver. Therefore, 1–2 mm of the long process of the incus must be resected. First, the incudo-stapedial joint is carefully separated. Then the distal part of the long process of the incus is separated using a laser. Finally, the mobility of stapes, malleus, and incus body is tested. All of them must be mobile. Adhesions should be removed.

Insertion of the Implant

First the PZT sensor is placed, using Glasscock stabilizers, in the superior edge of the mastoidectomy such that the tip of the PZT sensor can be positioned near and over the incus body. It is fixed by a first layer of cement. The tip is connected to the incus body by a microdrop of glassionomer cement, which, after drying, is separated from the incus. Thus, a 'neojoint' is created allowing free and unloaded movement of the incus while moving the tip of the PZT sensor. Then the driver is placed again, using a Glasscock stabilizer, in the inferior edge of the mastoid. Its tip comes through the posterior tympanotomy, touching, without loading, the stapes head. It should produce movements of the stapes in a direction vertical to the stapes footplate. It is fixed in the mastoid with cement and the tip is attached to the stapes head by a small amount of glassionomer cement. A final fixation of driver and sensor in the mastoid using additional cement ensures their stable position.

The sound processor and battery are positioned in the bone bed and fixed as described above. The cable links from the sensor and driver are cleaned and connected to the processor. Lastly, the system test is performed and, if satisfactory, the procedure is finished by suturing the muscle, subcutaneous, and skin layers. During surgery, the functioning of the implanted parts and their optimal positioning is measured using laser Doppler vibrometry. Before closure, a system test is performed.

Patient Experience

We have more than 10 years' experience with implantable hearing aids. Currently, we are implanting partially implantable systems and fully implantable systems in sensorineural and mixed hearing-loss cases. Since 2002, we have implanted 10 patients with the Envoy/Esteem I system: 7 within the international multicenter phase II trial and 3 with the same inclusion criteria after study closure. There was no surgical complication or early or late wound complications. There was no significant change in cochlear function as measured by bone conduction thresholds after the surgery. Nine of 10 patients achieved or exceeded their preoperative hearing results while enjoying the advantages of a fully implantable middle ear device. Two patients had transcanal revision surgeries to optimize the driver-stapes connection including 1 patient who was explanted after 12 months because of feedback. His stapes arch was high, and the tip of the driver touched the tympanic membrane causing feedback. One patient was explanted after 31 months of successful usage requiring processor replacement due to battery life depletion; however, he refused a new implant fearing further battery changes. Both patients had reconstruction of their ossicular chain with closure of the air bone gap within 10 dB between 0.5 and 4 kHz. One patient who continuously used the device on a 24-hour basis required a battery change after 28 months. Two more patients had battery changes after 37 and 39 months. The remaining patients use their Esteem between 3 and 40 months.

All patients implanted would make the same decision again, and two do not use their contralateral hearing aid any longer because of good benefit from the Esteem.

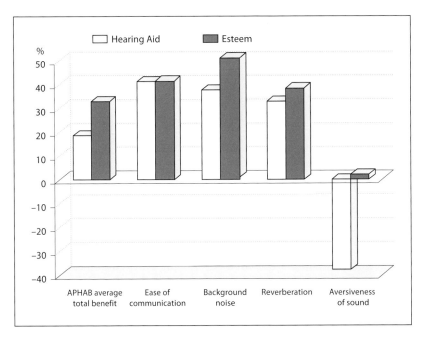

Fig. 3. APHAB results with hearing aids and Esteem system from 6 patients 3–6 months after the onset of the system. Ease of communication (EC): Communication under relatively favorable conditions. Background noise (BG): communication in settings with high background noise. Reverberation (RV): communication in reverberant rooms such as classrooms. Aversiveness (AV): unpleasantness of harsh environmental sound.

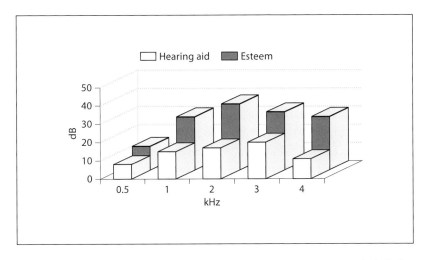

Fig. 4. Average functional gain with Esteem (dark bars) and hearing aids (light bars) 10–14 months after the onset of Esteem (n = 7).

Two wish to have their second ear implanted. The primary results of the Abbreviated Profile of Hearing Aid Benefit (APHAB) questionnaire for 6 patients are shown in figure 3. There was a considerable difference in functional gain with hearing aids and with the Esteem (fig. 4). Free field monosyllabic word recognition scores presented at 65 dB improved in all patients from a range of 70–90% correct with best-fitted hearing aids to a range of 90–100% correct with the Esteem.

Discussion

Conventional hearing aids, such as completely-in-the-canal hearing aids, are cosmetically acceptable but are appropriate only for mild-to-moderate sensorineural hearing loss. Therefore, cosmetically less acceptable behind-the-ear hearing aids are the option for the vast majority of patients. Conventional hearing aids require an ear mold, thus creating an occlusion effect. Ear molds are uncomfortable and, if the patient has a profound loss, there are often problems with feedback. The occlusion effect may be reduced by 'open ear' hearing aids, introduced in the last several years. Although conventional hearing aids have improved, they still have many deficiencies. Conventional hearing aids perform by overdriving the stapes. To do this, a column of air between the speaker and the tympanic membrane must move the ossicular chain. This is an ineffective method to amplify a severe-to-profound hearing loss, and requires a powerful hearing aid using a lot of battery power.

High- and low-pass filters, compression circuits, and other programmable features improve sound processing quality in newer hearing aids. However, many of these devices may still not perform adequately in noisy environments. The greatest problem with most hearing aids is poor quality and clarity of sound, particularly for patients with poor speech discrimination.

All hearing aid deficiencies can be overcome with a fully implantable hearing device such as the Esteem. In addition to reducing occlusion, feedback, stigma, and poor sound quality found in conventional hearing aids, a totally implantable device allows the patient to carry on with a normal lifestyle. The patient can shower, swim, scuba dive, or parachute out of an airplane. Patients of all ages are not handicapped during their activities. The system can be left on during sleep. Sweating during work or sports does not compromise system function. Patients can also walk through a strong electromagnetic field without worrying that their device will be affected. Its components have been developed and tested since the late 1990s [9–13].

Our preliminary results in a small series of a highly selected group of patients are more encouraging than the first results published from the phase I clinical trial [14]. Since then, the system has been improved in both technical and processing issues, and, with careful surgery, reliable results can be achieved. As with all new technology and surgical methods, there is a learning curve even for the experienced surgeon. The key to success with this system is the accurate positioning and fixation of the sensor

Maurer · Savvas

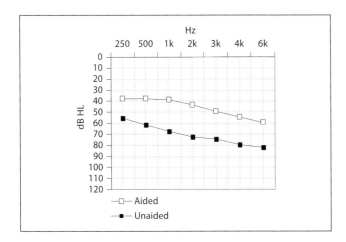

Fig. 3. Postoperative unaided and Carina-aided hearing thresholds in free field for 50 Carina users.

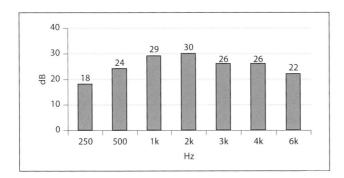

Fig. 4. Functional gain for 50 Carina users.

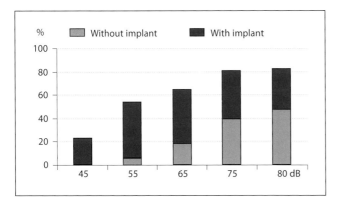

Fig. 5. Mean speech discrimination scores (binaural freefield Freiburg speech discrimination test with acoustically balanced monosyllables), aided with a Carina implant, of 50 users suffering from symmetric bilateral SNHL. Black bars = Aided with Carina implant; gray bars = unaided.

may fully recover after some weeks. The authors reported postoperative hearing gain with the activated implant. The sound quality was described to be better than suggested from the audiologic results.

General Indications for Totally Implantable MEIs

A general indication for totally implantable MEIs is the treatment of SNHL. This application is particularly useful when a patient cannot be fit with a conventional hearing aid. Conventional hearing aid use can lead to several problems in some patients, as listed below.

(1) Medically, earpieces can lead to intolerable
- occlusion,
- auditory canal inflammation, and
- difficult placement of the earpiece in the ear canal for patients with motor disorders of the hand.

(2) Audiologically, inadequate auditory rehabilitation can result if there is
- unmanageable acoustic feedback (whistling),
- intolerable distortion levels,
- a surpassing of the comfortable level, or
- inadequate speech comprehension, especially in occupational situations.

(3) Stigmatization refers not so much to aesthetics but rather to an actual, and sometimes significant, discrimination against a visibly handicapped individual, particularly in occupational settings. This may include the following:
- Discrimination at the workplace and when looking for work.
- In their private lives, individuals may also become socially withdrawn.

(4) Occupational reasons are important. In addition to reasons 1 through 3, which may contribute to occupational disabilities, difficulties experienced by specific occupational groups should also be considered. Doctors and nursing staff (stethoscopes), employees in call centers (ear plugs), and persons working in humid environments (the hearing aid falls out) may have additional difficulties with canal-occluding hearing aids. Working in places where heat and steam are produced may damage hearing aids. Persons with occupations involving sweating (hearing aids fall out), telephone work, speech communications (teachers, interpreters), or customer and negotiation-oriented services may not be successfully rehabilitated using hearing aids. When one or several reasons apply, rehabilitation with conventional hearing aids may be unsatisfying or even impossible in some patients. If specific indications apply, some affected individuals may now be helped using amplifying implants that are appropriate, adequate and indeed necessary.

Specific Indications

Each implant has its own specific audiologic indications that are described for each implant. Because partially implantable MEIs can provide acoustic advantages over conventional hearing aids, partially implantable implants are indicated for patients

Zenner · Rodriguez Jorge